ORGANIC

AROMATHERAPY

&

ESSENTIAL OILS

The Modern Guide to
All-Natural Health and Wellness

**ROCKRIDGE
PRESS**

Amber Robinson

Interior and Cover Designer: Regina Stadnik

Art Producer: Tom Hood

Editor: Rachel Feldman

Managing Editor: Van Van Cleave

Production Editor: Andrew Yackira

ISBN: Print 978-1-64611-402-3 | eBook 978-1-64611-403-0

R0

I dedicate this book to my firstborn son, Adler.
Adler was born with a congenital heart condition
that took him from this world at three weeks old.
His passing impacted my husband and I greatly
and instilled in our hearts a desire to live each day
doing what we love while making a difference; life
is too short and precious to live any other way.

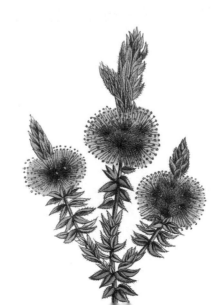

TABLE OF CONTENTS

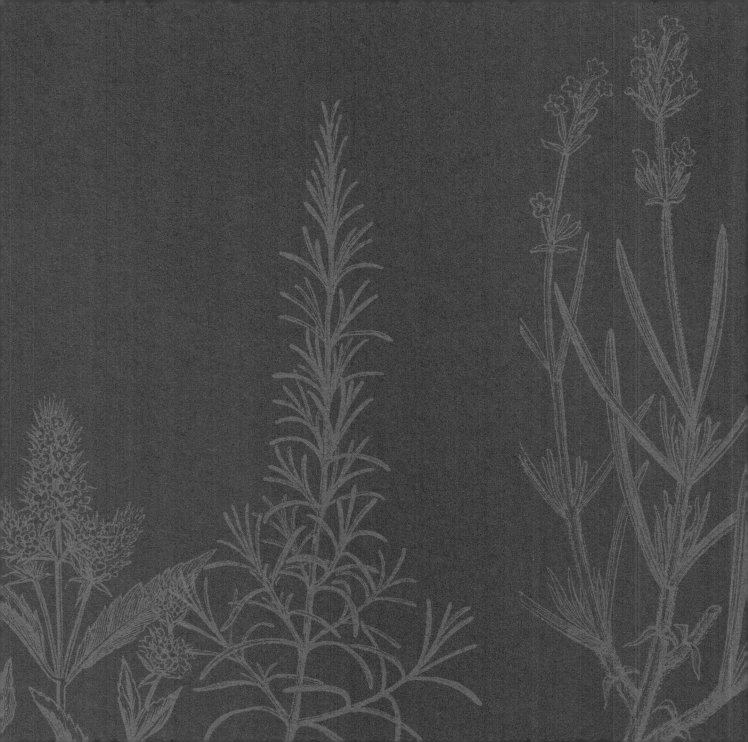

PART ONE

ONLY THE BEST FOR YOUR BODY

When it comes to finding credible information on organic essential oils, you may have noticed a glaring lack of resources available. The purpose of this book is to provide information on organic aromatherapy, as well as the many benefits organic essential oils can provide. Part 1 addresses how essential oils are made, why buying organic oils is the best choice, and tools you need to work with oils, along with detailed profiles on 50 amazing essential oils you can use in a variety of ways.

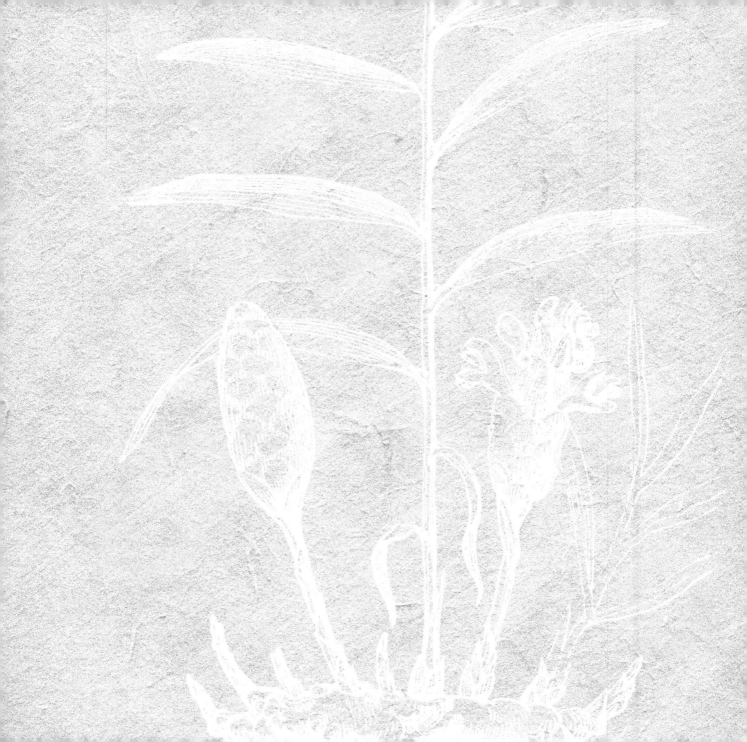

CHAPTER ONE

The Spirit of Aromatherapy

Most people have heard of essential oils but may not be familiar with how they are created, how they work, and how they are used. There is plenty of information when it comes to these topics—the problem is that there's too much. These days, we can perform a quick internet search and be inundated with a barrage of facts from various sources. At best, this can be overwhelming—at worst, deceptive or dangerous. In this chapter, I'll provide some clarity on what essential oils can do, how they're produced, and why it's so important to go organic.

INTRODUCING ORGANIC AROMATHERAPY

Essential oils are the aromatic compounds produced in plants that give them their unique scents, assist in pollination, and even work to naturally protect plants. When these volatile compounds are inhaled, they can play an important role in boosting the body's natural healing abilities. Aromatherapy is the practice of using essential oils to enrich our physical and mental well-being.

The actual term "aromatherapy" was not coined until 1937, but historians have discovered evidence that many ancient civilizations also practiced aromatherapy. Egyptians extracted plant oils for use during the mummification process, and the Greek physician Hippocrates discussed using aromatherapy in healing as early as 400 BCE. Burning aromatic plants to create incense is an ancient practice that has been well-documented in many different cultures.

Technological advancements have greatly changed the way in which essential oils are extracted from plants. Today's essential oils are highly concentrated plant isolates and are powerful and potent. Because of this, they offer a wide variety of benefits, ranging from emotional and mental well-being to household and personal care.

How Aromatherapy Works

Have you ever smelled something that automatically made you recall a past event? Perhaps a smell has reminded you of your childhood or past travels? When we smell something, the nerves in our nose send messages to our brain, and those messages help us determine whether a smell is pleasant. Our sense of smell is strongly tied to parts of our brain that store memory, so it's no wonder inhalation of concentrated plant oils can promote feelings of comfort or stress relief. Many plant oils also promote memory function: In a 2013 study, psychologists at Northumbria University found that sniffing rosemary essential oil enhanced memory function by as much as 75 percent. Due to their medicinal compounds, essential oils can affect other areas in the body when inhaled as well. For example, inhaling eucalyptus essential oil helps open the air passages in your lungs to make respiration easier when suffering from congestion.

The other way that aromatherapy works is through topical application, whether it is to soothe irritated skin, boost collagen production, or relieve cramping. Our skin is designed with barriers to keep the outside world from getting in. The amazing thing about essential oils is that they are capable of passing through these barriers and into the body due to their very tiny molecular weight. They also have both lipophilic and hydrophilic properties, meaning they can absorb into the layers of skin much easier than other materials. Factors that can help increase absorption of essential oils into the skin include warmth, the addition of carrier oils (more viscous oils absorb less), and how an essential oil was distilled (solvent extraction methods tend to produce more viscous oils).

Just one example: A 2017 study published by the National Center for Biotechnology Information proved that frankincense essential oil, when applied topically, significantly reduced the levels of two important inflammatory biomarkers.

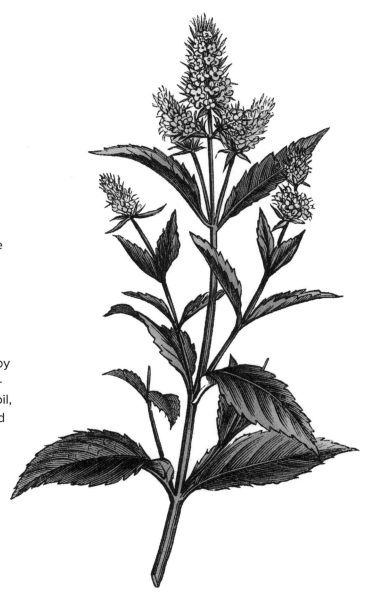

Aromatherapy: Ancient and Modern Medicine

Essential oils as we know them today are not quite the same as the essential oils used thousands of years ago. The first "essential oils" were likely plants infused in animal or vegetable fats and applied therapeutically. These oils were prized in ancient Egypt, China, and Greece. In ancient India, essential oils were used in Ayurvedic medicine as well.

Ancient Egyptians used aromatic oils and spices during the burial process, and ancient Greek physicians used aromatic plants in many ways to promote health and well-being.

With the advent of steam distillation around 1000 CE, essential oil potency changed. The oils used for perfumes and medicines became much stronger and more therapeutic. However, progress slowed down in the Middle Ages when the Catholic Church denounced the use of aromatic oils as being too decadent, even synonymous with witchcraft. Monks kept plant wisdom alive during this time, despite the risk of persecution.

By the end of the Middle Ages, essential oils slowly started coming back into popularity. In 1910, after discovering that lavender oil helped heal his burned hand, French chemist René-Maurice Gattefossé introduced the term "aromatherapy" with the publication of *Aromathérapie*. He went on to use essential oils during WWI to help treat wounded soldiers.

Another key player in modern aromatherapy is Dr. Robert Tisserand, a doctor who has devoted his life to studying essential oils. He published *The Art of Aromatherapy* in 1977, and spread awareness of how to use essential oils safely.

Since then, countless studies have been done to demonstrate the effectiveness of essential oils for a wide variety of ailments. For example, researchers have found that lavender essential oil does more than just heal wounds—it affects the human nervous system as well. In a 2013 study, the oil was more effective in the treatment of anxiety compared to a placebo (an inactive substance or preparation used as a control in an experiment to determine the effectiveness of a drug).

Scientists today have the technology to break down essential oils, identifying all of the constituents as well as how they act on the human body. As time progresses, we'll continue to discover more about the therapeutic effects of essential oils.

WHY GO ORGANIC?

If you were to sit down and list all the products you come into contact with on a daily basis, as well as what you put into your body, how many would contain only pure, organic ingredients? Household cleaners, makeup, lotions, shampoo, prescription medications, cell phone radiation, and our diet are all ways we come into contact with harmful chemicals and toxins each day. There have been very few studies on the long-term effects of exposure to these things. However, with cancer rates and autoimmune diseases skyrocketing, common sense dictates that whenever you can avoid exposure to these things, you should. As public awareness on the dangers of chemicals increases, interest in choosing food, household cleaners, cosmetics, and medicine that is organic is also increasing. Essential oils are no different.

Pesticides, herbicides, and fungicides are commonly sprayed on plants in the commercial farming industry and hailed as "safe and effective." However, research is emerging that shows the dangerous effects of chemicals once thought to be perfectly safe. In August 2018, a very large corporation was forced to pay $289 million in damages because its "safe and effective" herbicide was found to cause cancer.

Essential oils are concentrated plant material; depending on the plant, it can take anywhere from one ton to several pounds of dried plant material to get any measurable amount of essential oil. If you're using a nonorganic essential oil, that large amount of plant material has likely been sprayed with all sorts of chemicals—and you're inhaling a concentrated, highly potent amount of it.

While some nonorganic essential oil companies let the general public see their Gas Chromatograph/Mass Spectrometry (GC/MS) reports, many do not. This is most likely because these reports break down the oil into specific constituents and easily show whether adulteration or chemicals are present. What's more, many essential oil companies that have made these reports public do not use an independent laboratory to do the testing. The consumer is left to trust that the company conducting its own testing is being honest about purity.

This is why organic essential oils are rising so quickly in popularity. Consumers who choose organic oils can rest easy knowing they are avoiding exposure to harmful chemicals and possibly reducing the risk of long-term damage. That being said, it's important to educate yourself on what organic really means and how to ensure that you're getting what you're being promised. That's exactly what this book aims to help you with.

People, Plants, and Planet

When you buy organic, you are not only making a better choice for your body—you are making a better choice for the earth.

Mainstream agriculture practices often involve the use of pesticides. This is bad for us and the earth. When these pesticides are sprayed, they don't just kill the bugs causing issues for the crops—they kill everything. One of the most troubling issues with pesticides is that they kill beneficial pollinators like honeybees. Populations of honeybees are already dwindling, and if their existence is further threatened, food shortages may become a frightening reality.

When harmful chemicals are sprayed over acres of land, you can be sure they get into streams, rivers, and lakes. Even water treatment plants are not able to cleanse the water of all residual chemical substances. This impacts not only our water supply but also the various ecosystems living in the affected areas.

Organic farmers use natural fertilizers that both help plants grow and provide the soil with the nutrients required to maintain a healthy ecosystem. Buying organic means you could be positively impacting so much more than you realize.

FROM PLANT TO BOTTLE

So, what really goes into making that little bottle of oil? It all starts with the plant and how it's grown.

Organic Agriculture

Healthy soil is essential to growing the highest quality plants. Conventional farming methods rely on spraying or injecting the soil with chemical fertilizers. These synthetic fertilizers can actually harm the diversity of beneficial microscopic organisms normally found in soil.

Genetically modified organisms (GMOs) are another issue with conventional farming. Some plants have been genetically engineered to be more pest resistant, or produce bigger yields. This may sound great, but there are some drawbacks. For starters, nobody knows the long-term effects of GMO use since this is a fairly new practice. But what we do know is that when plants are modified to adapt to pests and diseases, those same pests and diseases can also evolve to become more powerful.

Organic agriculture ensures that the plants are not being synthetically altered. Organic farmers choose to avoid dangerous pesticides and herbicides, and instead use biological pest control methods. They choose to avoid synthetic and potentially harmful fertilizers and rely on natural alternatives like manure and compost. They also use ancient soil-nourishing techniques like crop rotation, composting, and mindful harvesting of the plants. These methods may be harder to employ, but hard work pays off with an ultrapure and untainted crop used to create essential oils.

Essential Oil Production

There are several methods used to create essential oils, including steam distillation, cold pressing, and solvent extraction. Some methods are better than others, depending on the plant.

Steam distillation, perfected by an Arabian alchemist named Avicenna around 1000 CE, involves heating water below the plant material to create steam that will travel up and collect the plant's essential oils. The steam recondenses and comes out the other end of the still in the form of hydrosol. After sitting for a while, the essential oils separate from the hydrosol. Related methods include hydro-distillation or a combination of hydro- and steam distillation. Since this process only involves heat and water, no adulteration or residual substances are left behind, just pure essential oils.

Solvent extraction is another way to get essential oils from a plant, especially when the plant cannot withstand the high temperatures used in steam distillation. Solvents used include petroleum, ether, methanol, ethanol, hexane, or CO_2. Many of these solvents can be found in the essential oil after the process is over, making this an undesirable method for those looking for completely pure, organic oils. Hypercritical carbon dioxide extraction of essential oils is one of the newest and best solvent methods because the process is able to remove most, if not all, of the CO_2.

Because many solvent methods can leave behind residue, make sure you carefully read the label to find out which method was used, keeping in mind that CO_2 extraction is often the best in terms of purity.

Cold-pressing is another way essential oils are obtained from plants. This method is especially popular for citrus fruits, where the peel or rind is used to collect oils. Cold-pressing involves using a machine to excoriate the surface of the rind to help release the essential oils. Next, the liquid is placed in a centrifuge to separate the oil from the liquid. The absence of heat may help prevent damage to any of the medicinal constituents of the oils, as well as help preserve the aromatic strength.

Top Benefits of Organic Aromatherapy

Promotes health without risk of long-term damage. Organic aromatherapy can be used as a natural alternative to (or in conjunction with) pharmaceuticals and western medical practices. You'll experience benefits to all aspects of your health, whether emotional, mental, or physical—without risk of chemical exposure or unpleasant side effects.

Truly natural alternative to synthetic products. Using organic essential oils ensures that you're replacing your toxic beauty and household products with an alternative that doesn't also contain pollutants. Plus—you and your home will smell incredible.

Better environmental footprint. Certified organic essential oils are made without harmful chemical fertilizers and pesticides that eventually make their way into rivers, streams, lakes, and other bodies of water. Organic farming employs more sustainable methods that benefit the soil and water in positive ways.

Stronger therapeutic effects. Organic essential oils are purer and thus superior in quality because they were not diluted with any unknown substances prior to distillation or extraction. This means that their therapeutic effects are unparalleled when compared to nonorganic oils.

Less risk of allergic reactions. Oftentimes, allergic reactions are caused by chemicals that exist in products. These chemicals range from synthetic fragrances to residual pesticides and herbicides. Because organic essential oils do not contain any harmful pesticides or herbicides, the chances of allergic or adverse reactions are much lower compared to nonorganic essential oil use.

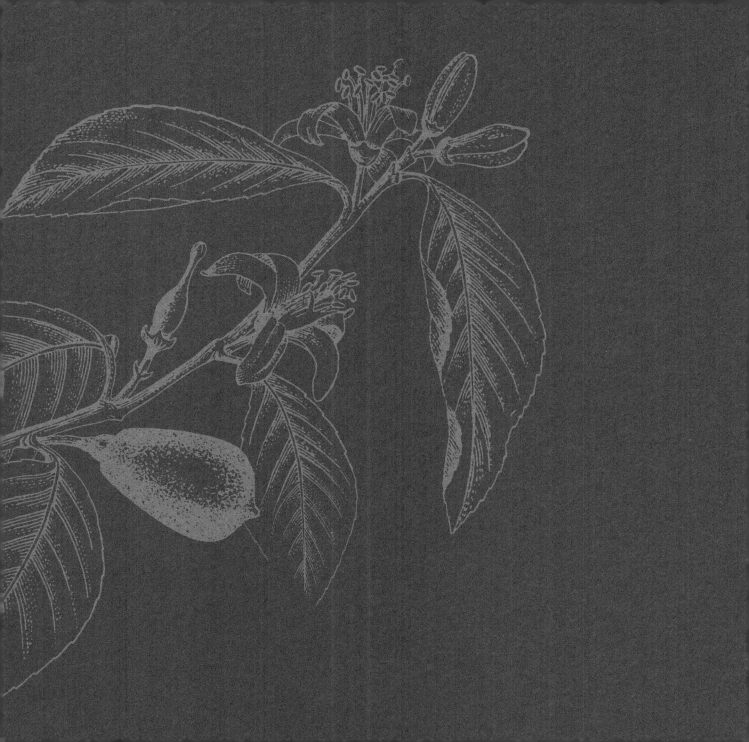

CHAPTER TWO

Your Organic Aromatherapy Toolkit

If you're new to aromatherapy, you're probably wondering where to start with everything that's available to buy online. And, with all the essential oil companies that claim to offer 100 percent pure essential oils, it can be extremely confusing trying to decide which company is the best. In this chapter, I'll tell you which organic brands to try, what to look for on labels, and which carrier oils you'll need. I'll also discuss the other tools and ingredients you'll need to get started. This chapter will give you all the information you need to shop like a pro!

SHOPPING FOR ORGANIC ESSENTIAL OILS

You may have heard that you should only buy essential oils that are "therapeutic grade" or essential oils that are "100 percent pure." There are many confusing marketing terms on labels that don't really mean much. Here are some key factors to keep in mind when shopping for authentic organic essential oils.

Where to Shop

As easy as it is to shop online, there are some things you need to know when shopping for essential oils.

Buy from a company website. If you choose to buy your essential oils online, consider buying from the company website rather than a large selling platform. Some large online stores that sell a variety of products also sell essential oils. However, these oils may be tampered with or adulterated. It is best to buy straight from the manufacturer when buying online to avoid the risk of receiving something that may be counterfeit.

Support small businesses. If possible, support small businesses that sell essential oils. In many towns and cities, there are stores that sell natural products. These stores are often authorized to sell various brands of essential oils as well.

Try stopping in and seeing what they have. Oftentimes, the owners are very knowledgeable and can help answer any questions you have about their oils.

Try popular organic shops. Plant Therapy is a popular brand of essential oil that allows small businesses to sell their oils. This company has a large line of USDA-certified organic essential oils to choose from as well. Mountain Rose Herbs not only sells organic herbs in bulk, but they also have a large line of organic essential oils that can easily be purchased from their website.

Ethical Sourcing

It's likely that a company that sells USDA-certified organic or sustainably/ethically wildcrafted oils will practice ethical sourcing, but it never hurts to do your homework.

For example, frankincense essential oil is created from the resin of the Boswellia tree. The most popular Boswellia species for essential oil use is *Boswellia carteri*. However, this tree was listed as threatened in 2008. If you are purchasing organic frankincense essential oil, try to find out where they are sourcing their resin. Are they growing the trees themselves? What are they doing to ensure this threatened tree is taken care of? The company you're buying from should be able to answer these kinds of questions.

Affordability

You may find that organic essential oils are slightly more expensive than nonorganic oils, but paying a little more for a superior, sustainable product is well worth it. Chapter 4 will give you a good idea of the prices of most organic essential oils. Some essential oils are more expensive due to their rarity and the labor needed to create them. Oils like jasmine and rose may be quite pricey for this reason, but you can get them at a reduced price by buying them prediluted. If the carrier oil used by the company is a good quality oil, these prediluted oils are perfectly fine to purchase!

Reading Labels

Reading labels can become very confusing when it seems like every label makes the same claim. All quality essential oil bottles should have the following information:

* Common name

* Latin name (genus and species, usually located beneath the common name or under the ingredients)

* Purity (100 percent pure if it is a single oil)

* Ingredients (there should only be a single essential oil or a blend of essential oils listed)

* Directions for use and safety information

Some other terms to look out for include:

Aromatherapy grade or therapeutic grade: One might assume that the term "100 percent therapeutic grade" on a label is significant. Unfortunately, this is a marketing term with no real certification value. Many of the companies using this term are certifying themselves with this distinction, although the average consumer may be led to think that a third party is giving out this illustrious "certification."

Purity: Another term that is thrown around a lot on labels is "100 percent pure." When reading labels, be aware that there is no official certification for this claim either. Any company can make the claim that their product is 100 percent pure, when it is not pure at all.

Organic certification: The United States Department of Agriculture does give out an organic certification. If you are looking for an organic essential oil, you will usually see "USDA Organic" somewhere on the label. Don't be too disappointed if you notice that the label does not say organic anywhere. Sometimes the plants used to create the oils are wildcrafted. Wildcrafted means that the plants were harvested in the wild, in their natural habitat. This means the plants were not cultivated or sprayed with pesticides. Mother Nature grew them, making them pure and high quality! Look for the term "wildcrafted" on the label.

Safety information: Another thing to look for on labels is safety information. Essential oil companies that are honest and reputable will always list safety information on the labels, as well as on their website. Look for information on proper dilution and use.

Natural, Nontoxic, Organic: Reading Between the Labels

Just because a label says the product is "natural" or "nontoxic" doesn't mean that it's organic. There is a rigorous certification process by the United States Department of Agriculture for any product that makes the claim that it is organic. Certified organic products are created in a more sustainable way that utilizes eco-friendly farming methods.

While any company can say their product comes from a natural source, companies that have certified organic products can take pride in the fact that their products come from plants that were not treated with pesticides or synthetic fertilizers. In this way, purchasing a certified organic product supports environmental conservation, sustainable farming practices, the survival and diversity of wildlife, and healthy water ecosystems.

Please also note that there are varying degrees of organic certifications. These include "100 Percent Organic," "Organic," "Certified Organic/USDA Organic" (for items up to 95% organic), and "Made with Organic _____" (for items up to 70% organic, with the organic components clearly listed).

Red Flags

Lack of safety information. When a company omits safety information on a label, it usually means they have not taken the time to consult with an aromatherapist on the safety of their products.

Clear or plastic bottles. Because essential oils can degrade easily with sunlight exposure, clear bottles should be avoided. Additionally, essential oils can damage or eat through plastic, so stay away from plastic bottles, too. The best quality essential oils will come packaged in amber or cobalt-blue glass bottles.

Too cheap. There is a fine balance between paying too little and paying too much for essential oils. If an oil is incredibly cheap, it may not be unadulterated. However, you can also overpay for oils, especially if you buy from a multilevel marketing company.

CARRIER OILS AND OTHER INGREDIENTS

Because of the potency associated with essential oils, carrier oils should always be utilized. This ensures that you are receiving a safe amount of essential oil and avoiding possible reactions. When it comes to creating your own blends and remedies, you will need to know which carrier oils will enhance the effectiveness of your therapeutic creations.

Carrier Oils

Carrier oils are vegetable-derived oils that come from the fatty portion of a plant. Many carrier oils come from seeds, nuts, or kernels. These oils are often cold-pressed and are not volatile, concentrated extracts like essential oils. Carrier oils are especially helpful for diluting essential oils and achieving a safe dermal application. Most carrier oils do not have a strong smell, making them ideal for diluting an essential oil while retaining its aromatic effects. In addition, there are organic versions of many carrier oils.

Here are some great carrier oils to consider:

Apricot kernel oil: This light carrier oil does not have a strong smell. It doesn't leave behind greasy residue and absorbs into the skin well. Safe for most skin types, this oil is a versatile base for many remedies.

Argan oil: This oil is a treat for the hair as well as the skin. It contains antioxidants and vitamins that help make hair shine and skin glow. This oil is a perfect base for skin and hair remedies.

Avocado oil: This carrier oil is a good choice for those wanting to provide the skin with more moisture. It is a very hydrating and replenishing oil best suited for dry, aging skin.

Castor oil: This is one of the thickest oils and one of the best emollients for the skin. A little of this skin-healing oil goes a long way, so it is best blended with another carrier oil to help thin it out.

Coconut oil: This oil is very thick but has so many therapeutic properties! It is naturally antifungal and can also help heal and protect damaged or dry skin. It makes a great base for creating ointments, salves, or balms. Always look for raw, unrefined coconut oil and avoid over-processed coconut oil called "fractionated" coconut oil, which possesses no real therapeutic value.

Grapeseed oil: This oil is very light in consistency. It makes a perfect base for those with acne-prone skin, as it will not clog pores. It can go rancid quickly, so always check the expiration date before purchasing.

Jojoba oil: Jojoba oil has the longest shelf life of any carrier oil. It is highly beneficial for the skin and can help restore and nourish. It is not overly thick in consistency, making it ideal as a base for skincare serums.

Olive oil: This common oil is a staple in many homes. It isn't just great in the kitchen; this oil is great for hair and skin. It doesn't leave behind a greasy residue and absorbs into the skin well. It is also easy to find in most stores. Look for organic extra-virgin olive oil.

Rosehip oil: This nourishing oil is full of antioxidants and vitamins. It is especially beneficial for aging skin, helping to promote balance and tone while preventing wrinkles.

Sweet almond oil: Sweet almond oil is very light and goes on easily, leaving behind no sticky residue. This is another great choice for oily or acne-prone skin. Like grapeseed, check the expiration date before purchasing to ensure it will last as long as you need it.

All carrier oils have an expiration date, and some expire faster than others. Remember to sniff your carrier oils from time to time, even before the expiration date, to check whether they have gone rancid. If they smell funny or off, it may be time to discard them. You can achieve a long shelf life by storing them in a dark, cool place out of sunlight and extreme temperatures.

Other Ingredients

Ingredients other than carrier oils are sometimes needed to create remedies with essential oils, especially cleaning products and cosmetics. Here are some useful and natural ingredients you may want to have on hand for the recipes in this book:

Alcohol: Don't underestimate the benefits of alcohol when creating recipes! There are two main types of alcohol: ethyl alcohol (vodka, rum, etc.) and isopropyl alcohol (rubbing alcohol). Both help kill bacteria and preserve recipes. Ethyl alcohol is okay for internal use, but isopropyl alcohol should never be taken internally. When purchasing ethyl alcohol, look for at least 80 proof. This type of alcohol is also available in an organic form. Isopropyl alcohol is not available in an organic form.

Aloe vera gel: This is simply the inner gel that comes from the leaves of the aloe vera plant. It is a wonderfully useful product because it is naturally anti-inflammatory and soothes the skin. It makes a wonderful base for skin-soothing oil blends. Look for organic, food-grade aloe vera gel, because it should not contain the preservatives that other types of aloe vera gel possess. Another option is to grow your own aloe vera plants (they are very easy to care for and need little maintenance). This way, you can take leaves and scoop out the gel as needed for remedies!

Baking soda: Also known as sodium bicarbonate, this common kitchen item is great for recipes that help get rid of unwanted odors. Several companies offer organic baking soda.

Beeswax: This natural substance created by bees helps thicken or harden mixtures to create lip balms, ointments, salves, and soaps. Purchase beeswax in pellet form, which is much easier to measure out for recipes.

Epsom salt: Comprised of magnesium sulfate, this useful salt makes a great base for bath soak blends. It naturally helps soothe sore, tired muscles. Look for Epsom salt that does not contain added substances like fragrances or herbs, so you can blend your own recipes.

Raw shea or cocoa butter: These ingredients add even more skin-nurturing properties to an oil-based lotion. Look for organic, raw, and unrefined versions of these butters.

Unscented liquid castile soap: There are several companies that make liquid castile soap containing organic and certified fair trade ingredients. In addition, some companies create castile soap that is completely biodegradable. This gentle, simple soap base can be used in cleaners, as a shampoo or body wash, and with pets.

Vinegar: Vinegar is a common household substance and also makes a great base for cleaners made with essential oils. There are two main types of vinegar: apple cider vinegar and white distilled vinegar. When purchasing vinegar, look for organic, unfiltered apple cider vinegar or organic distilled white vinegar.

Witch hazel: The bark and leaves from this tree have astringent and antibacterial properties. They have been used for years to soothe and treat wounds. Organic witch hazel can be purchased in extract form, and it makes a great base for various essential oil blends.

TOOLS AND EQUIPMENT

A number of tools may come in handy when making the recipes in this book. If you find that you love aromatherapy, some of the equipment listed below is not necessary, but is definitely nice to have at home.

Essential Tools and Supplies

Funnels: Tiny funnels make it easy to pour carrier oils into bottles.

Measuring spoons and cups: You will need a set of measuring cups and spoons in common sizes.

Mixing bowls: Some recipes will require mixing bowls. Use glass mixing bowls whenever possible.

Orifice removers: This device helps remove stubborn dropper lids and rollerball fitments. It can significantly reduce the chances of a spill when trying to remove these lids.

Pipettes: Pipettes are convenient for transferring essential oils into other bottles. They are long and help reduce the risk of spilling any precious oil.

Roller bottles: These bottles come in a variety of sizes to suit your needs, but the most popular size is a half ounce (15 ml). Purchase tinted bottles and avoid clear versions. Glass is always the best option, as essential oils can eat through plastic.

Spray bottles: Tinted glass spray bottles are great for any recipe where you need to create a mist effect. These come in a variety of sizes, but the two-ounce bottles are the most practical. Larger bottles may be more practical for cleaning recipes.

Storage jars and tins: Glass canning jars ranging from two to eight ounces in size are great for storing lotions, sugar scrubs, massage blends, and some cleaning blends. Two- and four-ounce tins are another option for lotions, salves, and scrubs. For oil blends and serums, one- and two-ounce tinted glass bottles are perfect.

Utensils: You will need some kitchen spoons for stirring and mixing. Choose wooden or metal utensils when working with essential oils; avoid all plastics.

Nice to Have Equipment

Inhaler: Inhalers are very reasonably priced, small devices that have a cotton wick inside. The idea is to drop the oils onto the wick, close the cap, and inhale the oils as needed. These make an excellent remedy on the go because they keep the necessary oils safely inside and are small enough to be carried in practically any size purse.

Ultrasonic diffuser: These are widely available and range from cheap to expensive. Don't think you have to spend a ton of money to get a quality diffuser—there are many dependable $20 to $35 diffusers available from online retailers. These small machines help vaporize water mixed with essential oils into the air so you can benefit therapeutically in your home.

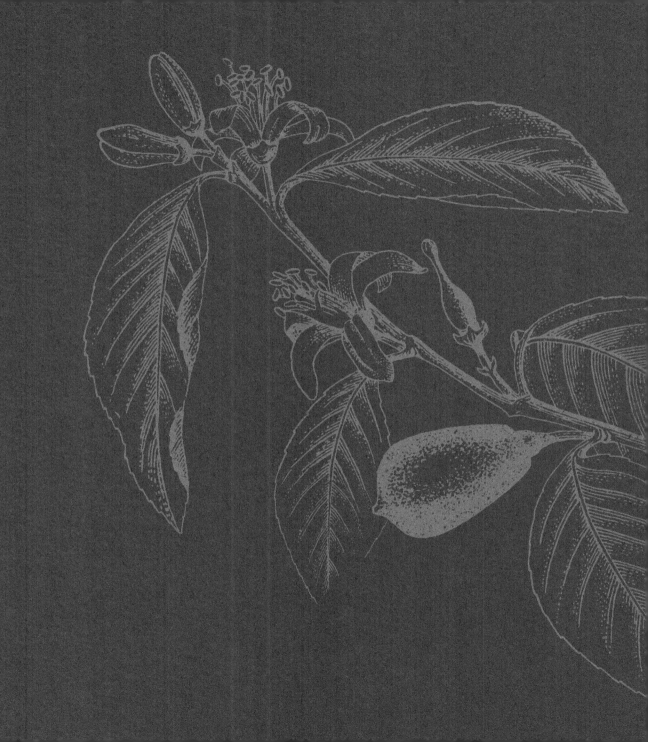

CHAPTER THREE

Using Organic Essential Oils

Essential oils contain volatile compounds and should be treated with respect. Improper use can result in sensitization or severe allergic reactions. In this chapter, you will learn how to use oils properly to get the most out of them. This chapter also includes safety guidelines to help you create remedies carefully.

METHODS OF APPLICATION

Aromatherapy is most effective and safe when applied topically or inhaled. There are several ways you can deliver the powerful healing effects of the oils to your body.

Baths/showers: Baths and showers are a comforting way to enjoy the benefits of essential oils. The steam created can help open pores and airways, and the heat can relax and calm the body. This combination makes the perfect environment for the addition of oils. See the PMS Bath Soak (page 87) for one way to enjoy essential oils in the bath.

Diffusers: Diffusers are an excellent way to inhale the healing properties of various essential oils. These machines create a mist or vapor with water and essential oils that can spread throughout a room. Depending on the oils used, diffusers can help purify the air and kill bacteria or pathogens that cause sickness. See the Virus Buster Diffusion Blend (page 110) for help purifying the air in your home.

Directly to skin: Essential oils can be combined with carrier oils and massaged into the skin on or near the affected areas. You can use your hands or a roller bottle to apply them. Massage is a relaxing and effective way to deliver oil blends to sore, tired muscles. See the Sore Muscles Massage Blend (page 102) for a recipe that can help provide relief for achy muscles.

Steam inhalation: Direct steam inhalation over a pot of hot water can open up clogged airways and provide almost immediate relief from sinus pressure, allergies, congestion, or colds. Try the Facial Steam for Healthy Skin (page 161) to see how oils can help the skin as well.

Other fun methods: Other valuable ways to deliver essential oils to the body include inhalers, aromatherapy jewelry, and compresses. Inhalers and jewelry allow you to directly inhale the beneficial aromas wherever you are! Inhalers can be carried in your purse or bag, and aromatherapy jewelry allows you to drop oils onto a porous surface to inhale throughout the day. Compresses can be applied topically for minor injuries like sprains. They can be applied warm or cold, depending on the issue.

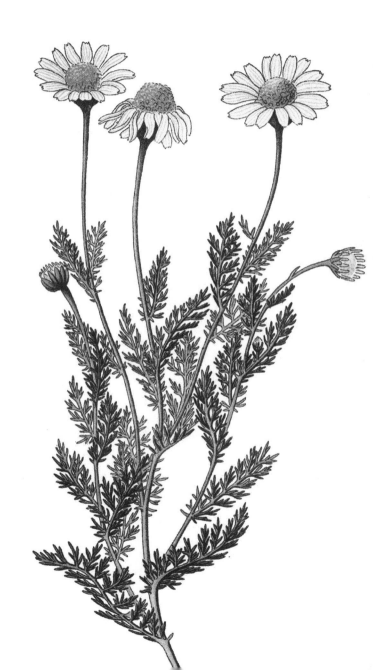

Best Blends for Every Season

SUMMER

Cool off on hot summer days with refreshing and invigorating essential oils. Use citrus essential oils to boost energy on those longer days.

Bergamot essential oil: Treat yourself to a relaxing spa day with bergamot essential oil. Use the Oily Skin Toner Spray (page 191) to enjoy its soothing benefits.

Lemon essential oil: Lemon essential oil is one of the most versatile essential oils there is. Use it to clean, boost your mood, or increase energy levels.

Lime essential oil: This citrus scent smells like the embodiment of summer! It can help provide physical and mental energy. It is also great for acne-prone skin that tends to flare up in the summer heat.

Peppermint essential oil: This oil provides a gentle chilling sensation. It is perfect for cooling off on hot summer days! Cooling Spray for Hot Days (page 108) uses this oil.

Tangerine essential oil: With a light and crisp citrus fragrance, this oil is sure to delight. Use it in a Skin Softening Sugar Scrub (page 166).

FALL

Fall is a time to find motivation to get started on new work projects or schooling, so oils that help motivate, improve memory, and reduce anxiety are perfect.

Rosemary essential oil: Proven to help improve brain function and memory, rosemary is a must-have to help with focus during cram sessions.

Valerian essential oil: Get a good night's rest with this relaxing essential oil. Valerian can help gently sedate overworked nerves. Try the Anxiety Inhalation Remedy (page 118).

Vetiver essential oil: Vetiver has an earthy aroma that is grounding. This oil is great for calming and focus. Try the Brain Fog Diffusion Blend (page 123).

Orange essential oil: One of the most uplifting oils, orange can promote a sense of positivity while also boosting energy and mood.

Cinnamon essential oil: This spicy oil can stimulate the senses, as well as kill unwelcome germs. It pairs well with clove, nutmeg, and vanilla absolute so you can create your own natural version of pumpkin spice—like Pumpkin Spice Perfume Spray (page 188).

WINTER

Viruses like influenza and colds seem to emerge during the winter months when our immune systems are bogged down. Warming and stimulating oils help kill pathogens, as well as create a cozy atmosphere in the home.

Clove essential oil: This oil can combat germs with its antimicrobial properties. Its warm, spicy scent is perfect for winter. Try the Virus Buster Diffusion Blend (page 110).

Ravensara essential oil: This essential oil pairs well with clove to effectively rid the home of germs.

Pine essential oil: This oil can help open airways when you are feeling congested and under the weather.

Frankincense essential oil: This grounding essential oil has a deep, earthy scent that combines well with other warm oils. It can help soothe dry winter skin as well. Check out the Wrinkle Reduction Facial Serum (page 163) for more of frankincense's benefits.

Eucalyptus essential oil: Breathe easily with eucalyptus essential oil. This oil helps open airways, ease pressure and pain, and provide relief from winter congestion.

SPRING

Spring is a time to celebrate life and the emergence of warmer, greener days. Floral essential oils help you embrace the season, while oils with antihistamine properties help control allergies.

Lavender essential oil: This floral scent doesn't just help calm the nerves; it also contains antihistamine properties that can help reduce the symptoms of allergies. Try the Allergy Buster Roller Remedy (page 70).

Tea tree essential oil: Tea tree oil is another great antihistamine. It can also help heal wounds, soothe irritated skin, and kill bacteria.

Jasmine essential oil: Celebrate the season with the gentle floral scent of jasmine. This ultrafeminine aroma can help boost confidence and sensuality.

Ylang-ylang essential oil: This bright and bloomy aroma uplifts and pairs fantastically with jasmine. For an effective combination of the two, try the Empowering Roller Blend (page 151).

Rose absolute: The mother of all floral scents, rose absolute can promote feelings of calm and peace. This beneficial oil is great for the skin as well. For a rosy recipe, try the Nourishing Makeup Remover (page 186).

USING SINGLE OILS

There are times when the use of a single essential oil is more beneficial than a blend. For instance, when using essential oils on children, single oils should be introduced first to avoid the confusion of trying to figure out which oil caused a reaction. This goes for inhalation and topical application. Essential oils should not be used at all on children under two years of age.

Another great time to use a single oil is if you have allergies. Using a single oil makes it very easy to figure out which oils you may react to and which are safe to use. After diluting properly, apply a tiny amount to a small area of your body to see if you are allergic to that particular oil. If you are especially allergic to a large variety of plants, you should probably avoid essential oils altogether.

Single oils are a good investment. They allow you to create your own blends depending on your specific needs—and your creativity.

As always, make sure to dilute any essential oil you are using before applying it topically. Not only is dilution necessary to prevent an adverse reaction, but it can also help the oil absorb into the skin better, thus increasing its therapeutic properties. The following page contains a chart to help you decide the proper dilution.

Diluting Your Oils

A glaring red flag is when someone tells you that it is okay to apply an essential oil neat. "Neat" refers to using the oil completely undiluted. An even bigger red flag is if you are told that a particular brand of oil is safe to use neat because it is the one true "100 percent pure" brand of oil and doesn't need dilution. The truth is that no matter the brand, no matter the extraction process, essential oils should *always* be diluted.

For starters, using undiluted essential oils quadruples your chances of having an allergic reaction. It is simply much safer to dilute these concentrated substances before applying them. According to essential oil researcher Dr. Robert Tisserand, dilution is very important in avoiding systemic toxicity, which can be less noticeable than skin reactions.

Proper dilution is also much more sustainable. The essential oil extraction process requires a great amount of plant material that is then condensed into a small amount of essential oil. To use essential oils neat is to promote unnecessary wastefulness.

A good rule of thumb for a 1 percent dilution is one drop of essential oil per teaspoon of carrier oil. This dilution is best for children. Here is a chart, based upon clinical aromatherapist Lea Jacobson's advice, that demonstrates how to achieve a specific dilution.

DILUTION	0.25%	0.50%	1%	2%	5%	10%
ESSENTIAL OIL AMOUNT	1 Drop	1 Drop	1 Drop	2 Drops	5 Drops	10 Drops
CARRIER OIL AMOUNT	1 TBSP + 1 TSP	2 TSP	1 TSP	1 TSP	1 TSP	1 TSP

MAKING YOUR OWN BLENDS

Since many essential oils work synergistically, combining certain oils in a blend can expedite and enhance the effectiveness of a remedy.

Creating targeted remedies and fragrant perfumes are two ways blends can be especially helpful. However, keep in mind that blends should follow safe dilution guidelines, especially when you are attempting to make a blend from scratch. For those who don't have much experience with blending, dilution, or identifying aromatic notes, make sure to follow recipes closely to avoid issues like a blend that doesn't smell "right" or a blend that causes skin irritation.

A Blending Formula

The great thing about blending is that you're able to create new and wonderful aromas. When combined, oils with certain base notes, middle notes, and top notes can create pleasant, balanced scents.

For instance, cinnamon oil is a base note. It pairs wonderfully with middle notes like nutmeg and clove, as well as a top note like orange. All together, these oils smell warm, gently spicy, and comforting.

Top notes: These are the first notes that can be detected in a blend. They volatilize (dissipate) rapidly. Examples of top notes include citrus essential oils like lemon, grapefruit, and orange.

Middle notes: These notes take a bit longer to be detected and are usually noticed after the top notes have dissipated. Essential oils like rosemary, thyme, and pine fall into this category.

Base notes: These notes linger much longer than the top and middle notes and can even last several days. Oils that are base notes have full, rich aromas, like frankincense, sandalwood, and myrrh.

STORAGE GUIDELINES

Essential oils do not last forever. In fact, most essential oils will begin to degrade after they are opened, and may last around a year, if that. Citrus essential oils have a notoriously low shelf life and usually last up to six months after opening.

The best thing you can do for your oils is to store them in the refrigerator. Oils will last much longer in cooler temperatures. You can double the shelf life of your oils by keeping them cold. Citrus oils may last up to one year after opening and other oils may last up to two years.

Occasionally, oils will demonstrate certain characteristics that will let you know if they are going bad. Oxidation happens when oxygen gets into the oils and causes them to degrade. Signs of oxidation include the oils becoming sticky or cloudy, or smelling "off." Also, watch for a decline in the strength of the aroma.

Keep the caps screwed on tight to help reduce the chances of oxidation. Also, take note of when you first opened a bottle so you have an idea of when it is due to expire.

For essential oil blends that use carrier oils, you can determine the shelf life of the blend by looking at the expiration date of whatever carrier oil you are using. Blends using aloe vera gel and/or distilled water can be stored for up to three years in the refrigerator. However, make sure to double-check the aloe vera gel expiration date just to be sure.

SAFETY GUIDELINES AND BEST PRACTICES

It has been said before but is certainly worth saying again: Just because essential oils are natural does not mean they are completely safe. Due to the concentrated nature of essential oils, side effects ranging from allergic reactions and skin irritations to drug interactions and contraindications can occur.

Whether the essential oils are organic or not, they are still potent substances that should be treated like medicine. Read on for safety guidelines to help you enjoy the benefits of essential oils while avoiding any potential harm.

Ingestion

Ingestion of essential oils is almost never necessary and can greatly increase the odds of a reaction occurring. Some dangers of ingesting include liver and kidney damage (due to the concentrated load of constituents that must go through each organ), as well as anaphylaxis, negative interactions with medications, and burning of the esophagus.

Dilution

Less is more. One drop of essential oil may not seem like much, but keep in mind that essential oils are extremely concentrated. For example, one drop of lemon essential oil is the equivalent of roughly one pound of lemons. Organic or not, overuse of any essential oil is not unlike overuse of a medication. Excessive use can have dangerous results.

Sensitivity

Know your allergies. Stay away from any essential oils that derive from plants or plant families that you're allergic to. If you're buying or making a blend, pay attention to all the ingredients listed. Any time you are concerned about an oil, perform a patch test with a small, diluted amount of the oil to ensure you are not going to have an allergic reaction. Avoid using multiple essential oils for multiple needs at the same time to prevent overexposure and sensitization.

Some oils are phototoxic. This means a reaction could occur on the skin if you apply the oil and then go out into the sun. Cold-pressed citrus essential oils like lime, lemon, bergamot, and grapefruit may have phototoxic properties. Avoid using citrus essential oils topically if you plan on going out in the sun for prolonged periods.

The body responds to shorter intervals of exposure when it comes to essential oil diffusion. In most cases, there is really no need to diffuse more than 10 to 20 minutes to enjoy the therapeutic benefits of the oils. This can also be said for topical application. Try to give your body tolerance breaks and avoid using the same essential oils over and over. Prolonged use could cause adverse effects.

Medication and Alcohol

Always consult with a medical professional before using essential oils if you are on any medication. Some essential oils can interfere with certain medications, especially topical hormone medications. In addition, never seek to replace a medication with an essential oil without consulting a medical professional.

Some essential oils also interact with alcohol. Clary sage can actually exacerbate the effects of alcohol, causing more pronounced feelings of drunkenness. Avoid using any essential oil while under the influence of alcohol or drugs.

Pregnancy

Because of the sensitive nature of the body when pregnant and nursing, consult with a healthcare professional before using any essential oil if you are pregnant or nursing. Essential oil use during pregnancy can increase your risk for skin irritation, as well as preterm labor. Avoid any essential oils until after the first trimester. Use half the recommended dosages of any essential oils while pregnant or nursing. Avoid strong oils that could negatively impact pregnancy, including but not limited to Spanish sage, vitex, fennel, rosemary, myrrh, yarrow, damiana, angelica, jasmine, basil, juniper, laurel, and lovage.

Children

Keep all essential oils away from children and pets. Just like medications, essential oils can cause serious issues if a child or pet touches or ingests them. If you suspect your child has come into contact with an essential oil, call poison control immediately.

Do not use essential oils topically on children under the age of two. For children under the age of ten, avoid any essential oils that contain the constituent 1,8-cineole (eucalyptol). These oils include rosemary, eucalyptus, wintergreen, oregano, ravensara, sage, and laurel. Peppermint, when properly diluted, can be used on children over the age of six. Check to make sure any oils you wish to use around children older than ten do not contain high amounts of 1,8-cineole. Never use more than two oils on a child at once.

CHAPTER FOUR

Your Go-To Organic Essential Oils

There are over 300 essential oils available on the market today. However, not all of these oils are organic. This chapter offers advice for building a collection, detailed profiles of the top 10 most useful organic essential oils, and a comparison chart for 40 more essential oils. All of the remedies in part 2 include these 50 essential oils, with the majority being from the top 10.

PEPPERMINT

Mentha piperita

Peppermint essential oil is most often steam distilled from the leaves and aerial parts of the plant. This highly aromatic member of the mint family can provide an instant cooling sensation, making it useful for reducing fevers or simply cooling off on a hot day. Due to its strongly aromatic nature, this oil also makes an excellent bug repellant. The invigorating and stimulating aroma of this oil can help boost energy and lift the spirits. Because of the tingly, cooling sensation the oil provides, it has been traditionally used in muscle rubs to help relieve pain. This highly versatile oil is also great for stomach issues, and helps relieve indigestion, nausea, and a sour stomach.

Safety Precautions: According to *Essential Oil Safety*, oils high in 1,8-cineole should be kept away from the face of any child under the age of ten. Peppermint contains this constituent, but in lesser amounts than some other oils. Therefore, it is advised to keep this away from the face of any child under the age of six.

Substitutes: Eucalyptus, rosemary, and spearmint (a great substitute if using on children)

Blends Well With: Rosemary, lemon, and lavender

Price: $8–$16

HEALING PROPERTIES

* Analgesic
* Antiseptic
* Carminative
* Cooling
* Decongestant
* Expectorant
* Febrifuge
* Insect repellant
* Stimulant
* Stomachic

Uses

Peppermint essential oil supports a healthy digestive system, helping relieve any digestive discomfort. It can also alleviate pain, reduce fevers, and boost energy. When properly diluted, it can bring relief to sore muscles when massaged into the skin. Because of its strong, minty aroma, it is great for opening the airways and reducing congestion.

* Dilute the oil by placing 1 drop in 1 teaspoon of carrier oil, then rubbing a small amount on your belly when you have digestion issues.

* Add 3 drops to an ultrasonic diffuser and run it for 10 to 20 minutes when you need an energy boost.

* To help with fevers, see the Fever Reduction Roller Blend (page 84).

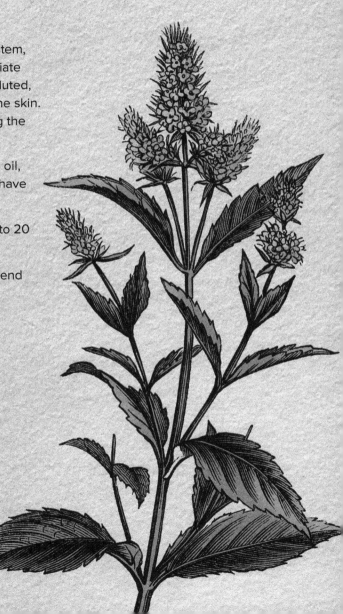

LAVENDER
Lavandula angustifolia

Lavender essential oil is most often created via steam distillation of the fragrant plant's buds and leaves, combining a lovely floral scent with an herbaceous fragrance for a truly unique aroma. This oil has many uses, for everything from treating irritated skin to soothing the mind and emotions. Because it is antimicrobial, it is a great choice for gently killing germs around the home or on the skin. It can be used to treat allergies and block histamine production. Its analgesic properties make it an extremely popular headache remedy among those who suffer from migraines or chronic headaches.

Safety Precautions: Lavender is one of the safest essential oils on the market. However, always follow the proper dilution guidelines when working with this oil.

Substitutes: Tea tree, chamomile, and geranium

Blends Well With: Tea tree, geranium, and rose

Price: $9–$16

HEALING PROPERTIES
* Analgesic
* Antidepressant
* Antifungal
* Anti-inflammatory
* Antiseptic
* Calming
* Carminative
* Insect repellant
* Nervine
* Sedative

Uses

Lavender essential oil can be used to lift the spirits, boost mood, and promote feelings of calm and peace, as well as reduce stress and anxiety. It is nourishing and soothing to the hair and skin and can help restore and treat minor irritations and wounds. Lavender essential oil is also an effective head-ache remedy by itself, or when combined with peppermint. Its antiseptic properties make it a great cleaning aid.

* Add 2 to 3 drops of lavender essential oil to ¼ cup distilled water in a spray bottle. Cap and shake vigorously, and spray on your yoga mat (or other objects around the home) to help gently disinfect.

* For an effective headache remedy, see the Headache Aid Roller Remedy (page 85).

* Place 3 to 4 drops in an ultrasonic diffuser and run for 10 to 20 minutes when you are in need of relaxation and peace.

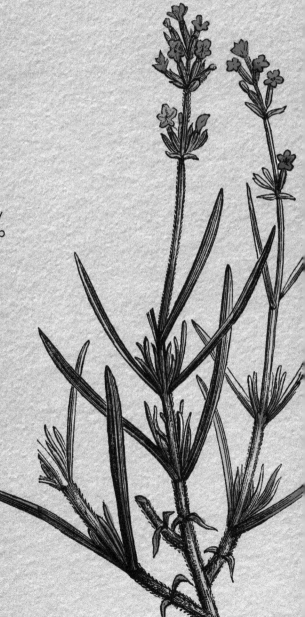

TEA TREE
Melaleuca alternifolia

Tea tree essential oil is created by steam distilling the leaves of the tea tree. It has a slightly spicy aroma. This oil has been used for years to disinfect and clean wounds, as well as promote skin healing. It can also be used to treat fungal issues like ringworm and athlete's foot. Because of its astringent and antibacterial properties, it is a popular natural remedy for treating acne.

Safety Precautions: There is a slight risk of dermal irritation when applying this oil topically. Make sure to follow proper dilution guidelines before using this oil to reduce this risk.

Substitutes: Lavender, oregano, and clove

Blends Well With: Lavender, eucalyptus, and lemon

Price: $9–$16

HEALING PROPERTIES

* Antibacterial
* Anti-inflammatory
* Anti-infectious
* Antifungal
* Antiseptic
* Antiviral
* Astringent
* Decongestant
* Insect repellant (especially lice)
* Sanitizing

Uses

Tea tree essential oil is often used to treat minor wounds like burns, cuts, scrapes, and lacerations. It can kill bacteria that lead to infection, as well as promote healing. Tea tree oil is great for treating acne and controlling oily skin. This oil is also an excellent remedy for athlete's foot and ringworm due to its antifungal qualities. It makes a promising treatment for sinus issues, especially sinus infections, because of its antiseptic properties. It can repel lice, so mixing one drop of it with one tablespoon of hair gel and applying to your hair can keep you protected.

* To treat a sinus infection, see the Sinus Pain and Pressure Roller Remedy (page 95).

* For help with acne breakouts and scarring, see the Acne Face Wash Remedy (page 158).

* Treat ringworm by blending 1 drop of tea tree and 1 drop of lavender with 1 teaspoon of carrier oil and applying a small amount to the affected area. Place a bandage over it to avoid rubbing the oils off. Reapply daily until the ringworm is gone. It should disappear in 2 to 3 days.

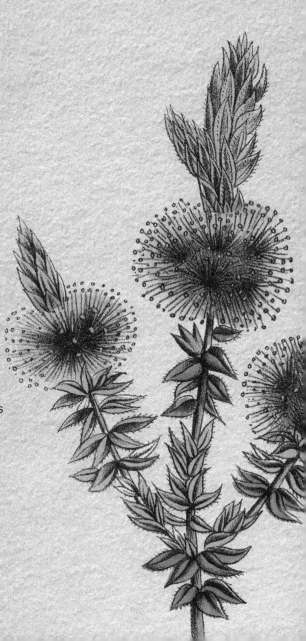

LEMON

Citrus limonum

There's nothing quite like the vibrant, uplifting aroma of lemon essential oil! Lemon essential oil is created by either cold pressing the peels of lemons or steam distilling them. This oil can instantly promote feelings of optimism and cheer. Not only does this oil help lift the spirits, but it also has powerful antibacterial and disinfectant properties, making it handy for cleaning. Lemon essential oil is also great for fighting colds and viruses due to its decongestant and antiviral properties.

Safety Precautions: This oil can cause skin irritation in people with sensitive skin. Follow proper dilution protocol when using it. Lemon essential oil is also phototoxic, so avoid using it if you will be going out into the sun.

Substitutes: Lime, orange, and bergamot

Blends Well With: Orange, grapefruit, and peppermint

Price: $10–$20

HEALING PROPERTIES

* Antibacterial
* Antidepressant
* Anti-infectious
* Antimicrobial
* Antiviral
* Carminative
* Disinfectant
* Febrifuge
* Hypotensive
* Insect repellant

Uses

Lemon essential oil can be used on the skin to treat acne, diffused throughout the home to fight viruses, or added to recipes to help clean the home. Inhalation of this oil can promote feelings of joy and positivity. When combined with ginger and peppermint, lemon essential oil can help treat digestive issues and nausea. It has gentle skin lightening properties that make it useful for fading scars or unwanted spots on the skin.

* Give your skin a healthy glow with the Skin Brightening Serum (page 180).

* Clean your home naturally using the All-Purpose Vinegar Cleaner (page 223).

* Lift your spirits with the Hope Restoration Diffusion Blend (page 137).

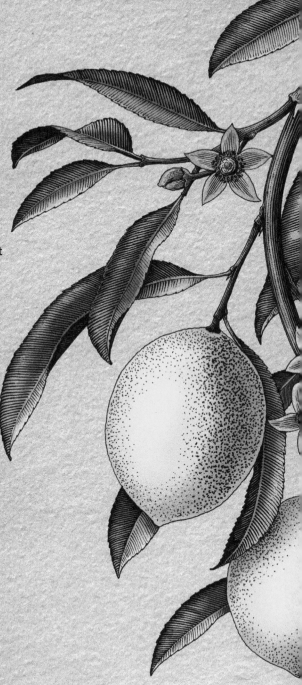

FRANKINCENSE
Boswellia carteri

The peaceful, earthy aroma of frankincense essential oil can bring groundedness and perspective. This essential oil is created by the hydro-distillation of frankincense resin. Frankincense is steeped in religious tradition. It is said to have been given as a gift to Jesus after his birth. It has been burned as incense for centuries and is strongly associated with spiritual enlightenment and progress.

Safety Precautions: Avoid using frankincense if the oil has oxidized, as it may increase the risk of skin sensitization or irritation.

Substitutes: Myrrh, patchouli, and cedarwood

Blends Well With: Patchouli, myrrh, and sandalwood

Price: $20–$50

HEALING PROPERTIES
* Antidepressant
* Anti-inflammatory
* Antiseptic
* Antitumoral
* Astringent
* Calming
* Carminative
* Expectorant
* Immunostimulant
* Sedative

Uses

Frankincense is a wonderfully anti-inflammatory oil and can be used to promote the healing of skin while creating a radiant and healthy complexion. Frankincense can also help heal scars and damage to the skin. It can be used to promote tranquility and serenity. It has been used traditionally to enhance spiritual connectivity. Diffuse frankincense to reduce stress and anxiety, as well as to calm the mind. Another great way to use frankincense is for respiratory issues, as it can help open the airways and rid the body of excess mucus.

* Try the Inflammation Buster Roller Blend (page 97) to reduce inflammatory reactions.

* Reduce stress and tension with the Tension from Stress Massage Blend (page 155).

* Achieve smoother skin with the Wrinkle Reduction Facial Serum (page 163).

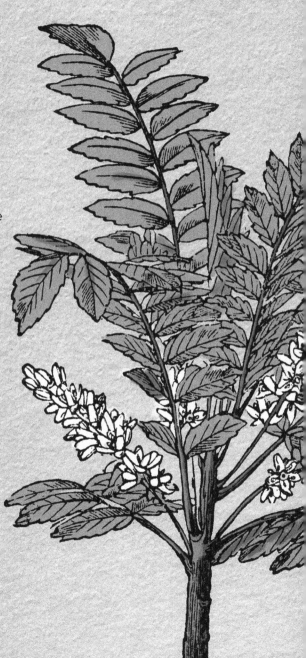

CLOVE
Syzygium aromaticum

Cloves have been sought after for thousands of years for their medicinal and culinary uses. Cloves are harvested from the flowering buds of the clove tree and then steam distilled to create the essential oil. The spicy, warm, and somewhat woody fragrance of this oil can be initially strong, but this is indicative of the powerful abilities of this oil to help with everything from pain to viruses.

Safety Precautions: Clove oil should be diluted to a dermal application of 0.5% because it can be irritating to the skin and mucous membranes. It may thin the blood, so avoid it if you have bleeding disorders. Do not take it with any blood-thinning medications. This oil is not recommended for children under the age of six.

Substitutes: Cinnamon, ravensara, and oregano

Blends Well With: Cinnamon, orange, and vanilla

Price: $10–$22

HEALING PROPERTIES

* Analgesic
* Anti-inflammatory
* Antimicrobial
* Antineuralgic
* Antioxidant
* Antiseptic
* Antispasmodic
* Bactericidal
* Carminative
* Hemostatic

Uses

Clove is an amazing essential oil for killing germs and bacteria that cause illness, and it can be used to sanitize areas you suspect may have been exposed to germs. Clove contains analgesic properties and has often been utilized to help with toothaches. It is a very strong aromatic oil and can repel unwanted insects. It may also ease digestive discomfort when diluted and rubbed onto the abdomen. Its powerful anti-inflammatory properties make it great for reducing inflammation in the body.

* Open up the sinuses and combat infection with the Sinus Pain and Pressure Inhalation Remedy (page 96).

* Promote oral health with the Healthy Mouth Rinse (page 194).

* If you are experiencing digestive woes, add 1 drop of clove essential oil to 2 tablespoons carrier oil and massage into the abdomen.

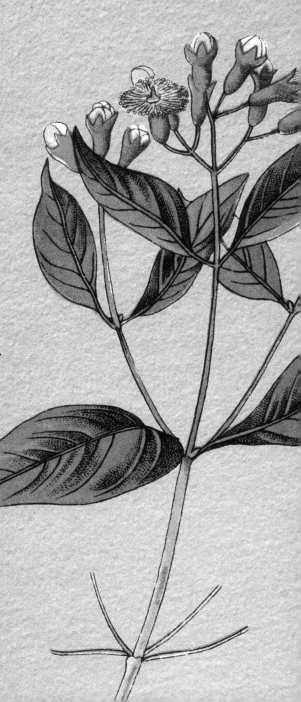

EUCALYPTUS
Eucalyptus globulus

The eucalyptus tree has been hailed as the "fever tree" and is native to Australia. The leaves of the tree are steam distilled to create eucalyptus essential oil. This highly camphorous oil has a menthol-like aroma that opens the airways and promotes respiratory health. In addition, this powerful oil can help fight infection and soothe pain. The versatility and effectiveness of this oil make it more than worthy of the top 10 list.

Safety Precautions: Eucalyptus oil contains higher amounts of the constituent 1,8-cineole. For this reason, it should not be used on children under the age of ten, as it could worsen respiratory issues. The maximum dermal application of this oil is 20%, so dilute accordingly.

Substitutes: Tea tree, peppermint, and wintergreen

Blends Well With: Peppermint, spearmint, and tea tree

Price: $9–$18

HEALING PROPERTIES
* Analgesic
* Antibacterial
* Anti-infectious
* Antiseptic
* Antiviral
* Decongestant
* Energizing
* Febrifuge
* Insect repellant
* Stimulant

Uses

Eucalyptus essential oil is one of the most effective essential oils for congestion, phlegm, and respiratory issues. It can be used to help clear the body of mucus and open the airways. Its strongly camphorous and analgesic nature makes it ideal for diluting and applying topically to sore, painful muscles. It can be diffused to rid the room of viruses and bacteria while relieving pain and pressure from blocked airways.

* Get rid of blocked airways with the Better Breathing Inhalation Blend (page 77).

* Alleviate sinus issues with the Sinus Pain and Pressure Roller Remedy (page 95).

* Add 2 to 3 drops to an ultrasonic diffuser to purify the air in a room after sickness in the household.

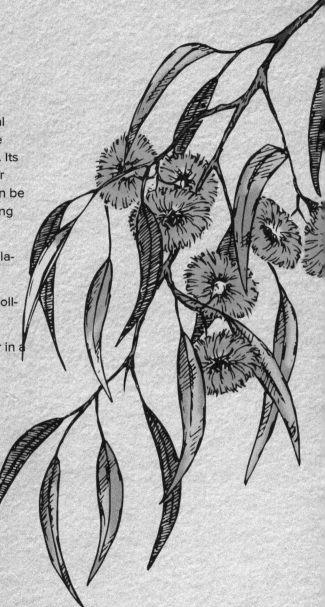

OREGANO
Origanum compactum

Oregano may be one of the most powerful essential oils available. It is created by steam distillation of the leaves and aerial parts of the common oregano herb. Oregano essential oil has a strongly herbaceous, antiseptic aroma. Oregano has a high phenol content, and while this contributes to its strong medicinal properties, it also means that you should exercise extreme caution when working with this oil. It can help treat everything from bronchitis to pneumonia.

Safety Precautions: There is a moderate risk of skin sensitization or mucous membrane irritation when using this oil. This oil should not be used around children under the age of ten. It should also be avoided if you are breastfeeding or pregnant. If you have sensitive skin, avoid using this oil topically. Avoid use of this oil in the bath, as this increases the risk for skin irritation. Never under any circumstances ingest this oil or put it in your ears.

Substitutes: Tea tree, eucalyptus, and ravensara

Blends Well With: Thyme, tea tree, and rosemary

Price: $12–$20

HEALING PROPERTIES
* Antibacterial
* Antifungal
* Anti-infectious
* Antimicrobial
* Antiparasitic
* Antiseptic
* Antiviral
* Decongestant
* Disinfectant
* Expectorant

Uses

Oregano essential oil can be used to fight viruses and bacteria that cause a wide range of issues in the body. Its antifungal properties make it useful for treating candida overgrowth and related issues. It can be diffused to boost the immune system during cold and flu season, as well as for cleaning and disinfecting surfaces around the home. This oil has even been shown to kill harmful bacteria like E. coli and salmonella.

* Fight back against viruses with the Virus Buster Diffusion Blend (page 110).

* Combat sinus issues with the Sinus Pain and Pressure Inhalation Remedy (page 96).

* If you are suffering from an ear infection and need relief, add 1 drop of oregano essential oil to 2 tablespoons of carrier oil and massage around the ear (do not get any inside the ear).

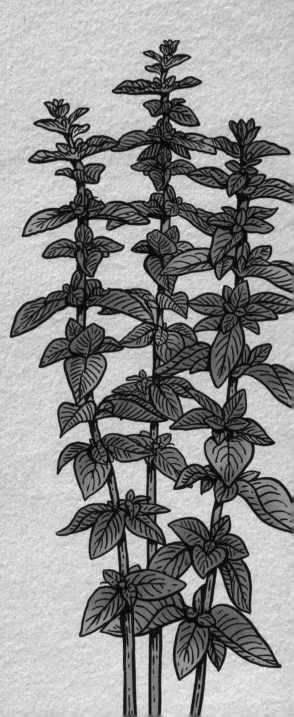

ROSEMARY

Rosmarinus officinalis

This sweet-smelling, herbaceous essential oil is invigorating and energizing. It is created by steam distilling the leaves of the common rosemary herb. This oil is said to promote a sense of alertness and focus. With a wide range of uses, rosemary essential oil is a staple for any top 10 list. From promoting circulation to improving brain health and memory, this essential oil does it all!

Safety Precautions: Rosemary essential oil can be potentially neurotoxic, depending on its camphor content. This oil should be properly diluted before using. Avoid using this oil on children under the age of ten years old, due to its 1,8-cineole content. Avoid using this oil while nursing, and check with a healthcare professional if you wish to use this oil while pregnant.

Substitutes: Oregano, eucalyptus, and tea tree

Blends Well With: Peppermint, thyme, and oregano

Price: $10–$18

HEALING PROPERTIES

* Analgesic
* Antibacterial
* Antifungal
* Anti-inflammatory
* Antiparasitic
* Antiseptic
* Astringent
* Carminative
* Hypertensive
* Stimulant

Uses

Rosemary essential oil can be used with other similar oils to fight viruses and kill bacteria. Inhalation of this oil has been shown to help improve memory by as much as 75 percent. It has been used traditionally to help with brain health and focus due to its stimulating and energizing properties. Rosemary can lift the mood and promote feelings of mental awareness. It works well in blends for digestive health as well.

* Treat minor bruises with the Bruise Roller Blend (page 72).

* Improve your memory with the Enhanced Memory Inhalation Blend (page 142).

* Because rosemary helps with circulation, add 1 or 2 drops to 2 tablespoons castor oil and use a small amount on hair to treat hair loss or a receding hairline. Apply a small amount to the hair and gently massage it into the scalp. Let it sit for 10 minutes before rinsing. Do this up to three times weekly.

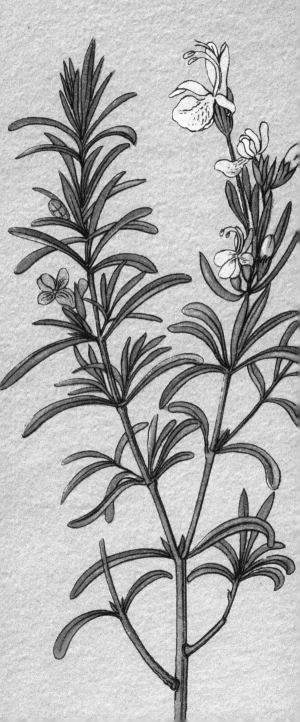

CHAMOMILE

Matricaria recutita, Chamaemelum nobile

Chamomile, with its light, fruity, and floral aroma, puts the mind at ease and promotes a sense of calm and serenity. This essential oil is created by steam distilling the flowering heads of the plant. There are two common kinds of chamomile: Roman and German chamomile. Both have very similar therapeutic properties. One difference between the two oils is that German chamomile essential oil is a dark blue color due to the sesquiterpene called chamazulene. Chamomile is known for its gentle sedative abilities, as well as for its antispasmodic and analgesic properties.

Safety Precautions: Drug interactions may occur if you are using drugs metabolized by CYP2D6 along with chamomile essential oil, including tricyclic antidepressants, psychotherapeutic drugs, codeine, and Tamoxifen. Avoid chamomile if you have allergies to plants in any related family, such as artichoke, aster, dahlia, dandelion, marigold, ragweed, sunflower, or yarrow.

Substitutes: Lavender, vetiver, and clary sage

Blends Well With: Lavender, patchouli, and clary sage

Price: $35–$50

HEALING PROPERTIES

* Analgesic
* Anti-allergenic
* Anti-inflammatory
* Antiphlogistic
* Antispasmodic
* Bactericidal
* Carminative
* Digestive
* Sedative
* Stomachic

Uses

Due to its antispasmodic and skin-soothing properties, chamomile essential oil makes a great addition to a muscle rub for muscle spasms and twitches. It can also help soothe dry, irritated skin in need of nourishment. Chamomile is a great remedy for digestive complaints and can be applied in a carrier oil to the abdomen for massage. The calming aroma of this oil makes it ideal for promoting relaxation while alleviating stress, anxiety, and frustration.

* Soothe sunburned skin with Sunburn Remedy Spray (page 109).

* Take advantage of chamomile's antispasmodic properties with the Restless Leg Spray Blend (page 101).

* Unwind with the Long Day Bath Soak for Stress and Tension Relief (page 154).

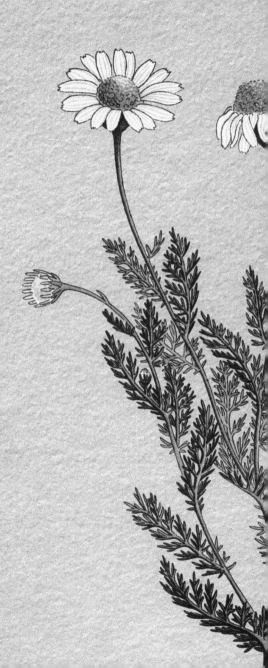

ESSENTIAL OIL	PRICE	SAFETY PRECAUTIONS	SUBSTITUTES	USES
BASIL	$8	Ages 8+	Tea Tree	Antibacterial, Astringent, Skin and Hair Care
BERGAMOT	$17	Ages 5+	Lavender, Chamomile, Tangerine	Mood Elevation, Mental/Emotional Well-being, Soothing, Oil Control
BIRCH	$10	Ages 10+	Copaiba, Peppermint	Pain Relief, Antibacterial, Antifungal
BLACK PEPPER	$15	Ages 10+	Wintergreen, Peppermint, Rosemary	Stimulating, Invigorating, Warming
CAJEPUT	$7	Ages 10+	Cinnamon, Clove, Ravensara	Antibacterial, Calming, Decongestant
CARDAMOM	$20	Ages 10+	Chamomile, Lavender	Antiseptic, Antimicrobial, Digestive Health
CEDARWOOD	$7	Ages 5+	Sandalwood, Frankincense, Vetiver	Calming, Grounding, Respiratory Aid
CINNAMON	$9	Ages 10+	Clove, Ravensara	Antiviral, Decongestant
CITRONELLA	$5	Ages 6+	Lemongrass	Uplifting, Energizing, Bug Repellant
CLARY SAGE	$18	Ages 15+ Avoid use with alcohol	Lavender, Chamomile	Sedative, Pain Relief, Antispasmodic, Uterine Tonic
COPAIBA	$8	Ages 10+	Clove	Pain Relieving, Respiratory Aid, Calming, Warming
CYPRESS	$15	Ages 10+	Frankincense	Skin Healing, Scar Fading, Grounding

ESSENTIAL OIL	PRICE	SAFETY PRECAUTIONS	SUBSTITUTES	USES
GERANIUM	$20	Ages 6+	Lavender, Ylang-Ylang, Rose Absolute	Skin-Soothing, Calming, Mood Elevation
GINGER	$20	Ages 6+	Rosemary, Lemon, Peppermint	Anti-Inflammatory, Digestive Health, Anti-Nausea
GRAPEFRUIT	$10	Ages 10+ Potentially phototoxic	Orange, Lemon, Lime	Energizing, Mood Elevation, Antioxidant
HELICHRYSUM	$35	Ages 6+	Lavender, Geranium	Skin-Healing, Anti-Inflammatory, Soothing
JASMINE	$50	Ages 15+	Geranium, Lavender, Ylang-Ylang	Boosting Feminine Confidence, Uplifting, Aphrodisiac
LEMONGRASS	$6	Ages 8+	Citronella, Lemon	Bug Repellant, Blood Pressure, Mood Elevation
LIME	$10	Ages 8+ Potentially phototoxic	Lemon	Energizing, Mood Elevation, Stimulating
MARJORAM	$12	Ages 10+	Eucalyptus, Chamomile	Antispasmodic, Antiviral, Antiseptic, Pain Relieving
MELISSA	$40	Ages 8+	Ravensara, Cinnamon, Clove, Marjoram	Antiviral, Uplifting, Energizing
MYRRH	$40	Ages 10+ Not recommended during pregnancy	Frankincense, Patchouli, Sandalwood	Grounding, Calming, Antibacterial, Anti-Inflammatory

Continued

ESSENTIAL OIL	PRICE	SAFETY PRECAUTIONS	SUBSTITUTES	USES
NEROLI	$50	Ages 6+	Orange, Bergamot	Uplifting, Balancing, Sedative, Digestive Health, Antibacterial
NUTMEG	$12	Ages 10+ Carcinogenic in high doses	Clove	Pain Relief, Energizing, Uplifting
ORANGE	$8	Ages 5+	Lemon, Tangerine	Mood Elevation, Energy Boost, Disinfectant
PATCHOULI	$12	Ages 6+	Myrrh, Sandalwood, Frankincense, Cedarwood	Balancing, Skin-Soothing, Grounding, Calming
PETITGRAIN	$10	Ages 6+	Patchouli, Frankincense	Sedative, Skin-Soothing
PINE	$10	Ages 5+	Cedarwood, Peppermint, Eucalyptus	Decongestant, Pain Relief
RAVENSARA	$20	Ages 10+	Cinnamon, Clove, Oregano	Antiviral, Antibacterial
ROSE ABSOLUTE	$40	Ages 6+	Lavender, Ylang-Ylang, Jasmine	Astringent, Skin-Soothing, Balancing
SANDALWOOD	$25	Ages 8+	Cedarwood, Frankincense, Patchouli	Grounding, Skin-Soothing, Calming, Aphrodisiac
SPEARMINT	$8	Ages 5+	Peppermint	Anti-Nausea, Digestive Health, Invigorating
TANGERINE	$10	Ages 8+	Orange	Uplifting, Invigorating, Stimulating

ESSENTIAL OIL	PRICE	SAFETY PRECAUTIONS	SUBSTITUTES	USES
THYME	$13	Ages 10+	Oregano	Antiseptic, Antimicrobial, Antiviral
VALERIAN	$30	Ages 10+	Chamomile, Lavender, Sandalwood	Sedative, Sleep Aid, Calming
VANILLA ABSOLUTE	$40	Ages 5+	Cinnamon	Warming, Calming
VETIVER	$35	Ages 5+	Frankincense, Cedarwood, Patchouli	Calming, Grounding, Focus
VITEX	$40	Ages 16+	Jasmine, Ylang-Ylang	Hormone Balance, Emotional Well-being, Fertility
WINTERGREEN	$10	Ages 10+ Can be irritating to mucous membranes	Peppermint, Eucalyptus	Warming, Stimulating, Pain Relieving
YLANG-YLANG	$15	Ages 10+	Jasmine, Lavender	Calming, Uplifting, Skin-Soothing

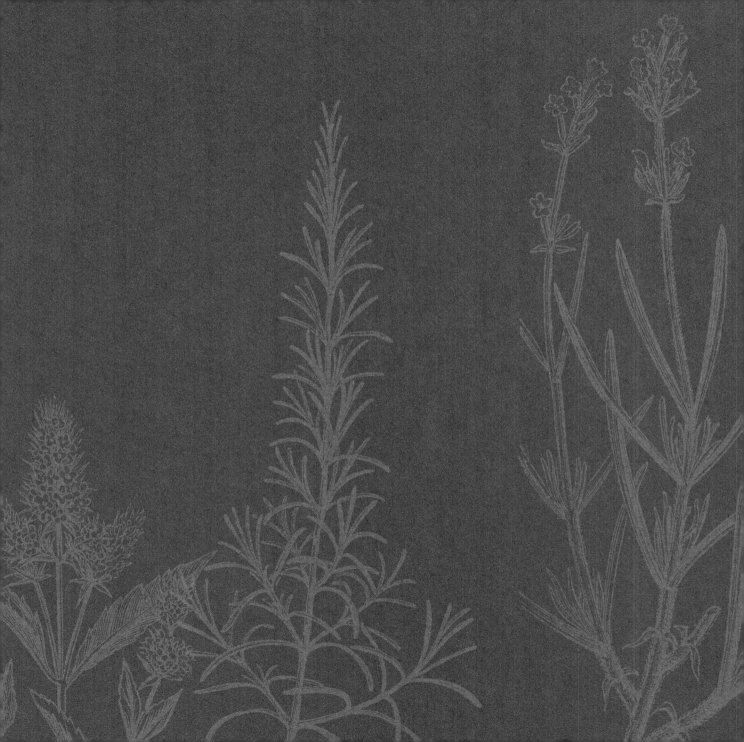

PART TWO

ORGANIC REMEDIES FOR EVERYDAY LIVING

This section offers a range of 150 organic remedies for natural wellness in several categories: Health and Everyday Ailments, Emotional and Mental Well-being, Cosmetics and Personal Care, and Home and Outdoors. All of the oils in these recipes were profiled in part 1. Each chapter is organized A to Z by ailment.

CHAPTER FIVE

Everyday Health and Ailments

The therapeutic effects of essential oils are truly amazing. They provide us with a natural way to stay healthy and can replace a number of over-the-counter medications, ointments, and pills. From opening the airways during times of congestion and combating viruses, to relieving headaches and soothing sore, tired muscles, essential oils get the job done. Not only are these oils effective, but they also provide the added benefit of a natural alternative to other products packed with toxic substances.

ALLERGY BUSTER ROLLER REMEDY

Topical ✳ *Safe for ages 10+*

This blend aims to combat the causes, as well as the symptoms, of common airborne allergies like pollen, dust, mold, and pet dander. The combination of antihistamine, anti-inflammatory, antispasmodic, and soothing oils in this blend work synergistically to help with allergy symptoms.

10 drops tea tree

10 drops lavender

6 drops lemongrass

5 drops sandalwood

5 drops peppermint

1 tablespoon carrier oil of choice

———

½-ounce (15 ml) tinted glass
   roller bottle

5 pipettes

1 small funnel

1. Add the essential oils to the roller bottle using pipettes.

2. Using the funnel, fill the bottle with the carrier oil. Place the roller and cap on the bottle and shake well.

3. Apply a small amount to the inside of the wrists and bring your hands up to your face to inhale deeply for allergy relief and to help open the airways. You can also apply the roller to your chest and massage the oil in completely as needed for allergy relief.

ALLERGY INHALATION REMEDY

Direct Inhalation ✳ *Safe for ages 10+*

This powerful combination of essential oils works together to block histamine production, clear the sinuses, and prevent infection. It may also kill bacteria and prevent sinus infections caused by excess mucus.

5 drops tea tree

3 drops peppermint

2 drops oregano

2 drops thyme

———

1 aromatherapy inhaler

4 pipettes

Place the essential oils onto the cotton wick of the inhaler using pipettes. Snap the cap firmly into place. When you feel the symptoms of allergies coming on, take 3 to 5 deep breaths of the inhaler every 15 minutes, as needed.

TIP: *It is best to take this inhaler with you on the go, because you never know when you might come into contact with an environment that may upset your allergies.*

BRUISE ROLLER BLEND

Topical ✷ *Safe for ages 10+*

Bruises can result in soreness, accompanied by various shades of discoloration that can be bothersome. This blend can reduce inflammation, promote circulation, and help with tenderness and achiness in the area.

5 drops lavender

4 drops helichrysum

4 drops frankincense

3 drops rosemary

1 tablespoon jojoba oil

———

½-ounce (15 ml) tinted glass
  roller bottle

1 small funnel

4 pipettes

1. Add the essential oils to the roller bottle using pipettes.

2. Place the funnel on the bottle and fill with the jojoba oil. Place the roller and cap on the bottle and shake well.

3. Apply to the fingertips and then massage gently into bruised areas of the body. Repeat up to twice daily.

BURN CARE COMPRESS REMEDY

Topical ✳ Safe for ages 6+

Soothing antimicrobial and anti-inflammatory essential oils pair up to promote healing and tissue regeneration. This method of application can be cooling and calming to skin that has experienced recent trauma. This recipe is best for mild to moderate burns where there are no exposed layers of skin.

1 cup distilled water

5 drops lavender

5 drops tea tree

—————

16-ounce canning jar with lid

1. Fill the jar with the cool distilled water.

2. Add the essential oils to the water. Secure the lid tightly and vigorously shake the contents.

3. Immediately place a small cloth in the container to soak up the contents of the container. Wring the cloth out into the jar.

4. Apply the cloth to the area and leave it on for 30 minutes. Repeat this up to five times daily (always shake vigorously before placing the cloth into the container) to promote healing and pain relief.

TIP: *Aloe vera is another amazing burn remedy that can be directly applied to the affected area in between compress treatments. Simply apply food-grade aloe vera gel or the insides of an aloe vera houseplant leaf to the burn.*

CIRCULATION MASSAGE BLEND

Topical ✳ *Safe for ages 10+*

Poor circulation may cause numbness or purple- and blue-tinted extremities. To promote circulation, this recipe combines warming and stimulating essential oils.

4 drops rosemary

4 drops black pepper

2 drops wintergreen

1 drop cinnamon

1 drop clove

2 tablespoons carrier oil
  of choice

————

1-ounce tinted glass bottle
  with lid

5 pipettes

1 small funnel

1. Add the essential oils to the bottle using pipettes.

2. Using the funnel, fill the bottle with the carrier oil. Secure the lid on the bottle and shake gently to blend.

3. Massage a small amount of this oil into the affected areas until it is fully absorbed into the skin. Apply up to twice a day to promote circulation. Avoid getting this oil blend in open wounds.

BLOOD PRESSURE HELP ROLLER BLEND

Topical ✳ Safe for ages 10+

This blend combines an oil to calm the mind and body with an oil that has been proven to help lower blood pressure. Together, they make a great combination for stressful situations.

3 drops melissa

3 drops lemongrass

1 tablespoon carrier oil of choice

———

½-ounce (15 ml) tinted glass
   roller bottle

2 pipettes

1 small funnel

1. Add the essential oils to the container using pipettes.

2. Using the funnel, fill the bottle with the carrier oil. Place the roller and cap on the bottle and shake gently to blend.

3. Apply a small amount on the back of the neck and pulse points during stressful situations to calm the body and mind.

COUGH AND CONGESTION CHEST RUB BLEND

Topical ✻ *Safe for ages 10+*

The oils in this blend work together to help break up congestion and mucus that has settled in the chest. This combination of oils has warming, antimicrobial, and anti-inflammatory properties that can target the stuffiness, inflammation, and pain associated with chest congestion.

5 drops pine

4 drops cedarwood

3 drops cajeput

3 drops orange

2 drops eucalyptus

2 tablespoons carrier oil
of choice

———

1-ounce tinted glass bottle
with lid

5 pipettes

1 small funnel

1. Add the essential oils to the bottle using pipettes.

2. Using the funnel, fill the bottle with the carrier oil. Secure the lid on the bottle and shake well.

3. Dip your finger into the jar and massage a small amount onto the chest area when you are suffering from congestion or a cough.

4. It is best to apply this blend while you are lying down. Massage in a circular motion over your chest until the oil has absorbed into the skin. Take deep breaths and inhale the airway-opening aromas. Do this as needed for cough and congestion, up to three times daily.

TIP: *It is best to apply the blend while you are lying down, as massage blends can drip and run if applied while standing.*

BETTER BREATHING INHALATION BLEND

Direct Inhalation ✻ *Safe for ages 10+*

This inhalation blend is for opening airways and promoting better breathing while congested. Powerful aromatic oils like eucalyptus and pine work to open the respiratory passages, while soothing geranium reduces coughing. Perhaps the most powerful of all, oregano is highly antimicrobial and can fight infection in the sinuses and airways.

5 drops eucalyptus

5 drops pine

4 drops geranium

3 drops oregano

1 aromatherapy inhaler

4 pipettes

Place the essential oils onto the cotton wick of the inhaler using pipettes. Snap the cap firmly into place. Take several deep breaths from the inhaler and wait 10 minutes before repeating, if necessary.

CHILDREN'S COUGH AND CONGESTION ROLLER BLEND

Topical ✻ *Safe for ages 5+*

It is best to keep remedies as simple as possible for children and to choose oils that are gentle and effective. Orange oil eases inflammation and cedarwood is great for fighting bacteria and relieving pain. Both oils are also soothing, making them great choices for kids. Cedarwood is also comforting and calming, helping little ones sleep better when suffering from congestion.

3 drops cedarwood

3 drops orange

1 tablespoon carrier oil of choice

———

½-ounce (15 ml) tinted glass roller bottle

2 pipettes

1 small funnel

1. Add the essential oils to the roller bottle using pipettes.

2. Using the funnel, fill the bottle with the carrier oil. Place the roller and cap on the bottle and shake well.

3. Apply a small amount in a circular pattern to the chest and then massage it into the chest completely until it has absorbed into the skin.

TIP: *Make sure the carrier oil you choose is not too thick (like castor oil) or it may not come out of the rollerball very well.*

NIX NAUSEA ROLLER BLEND

Topical ✳ *Safe for ages 6+*

A blend of fresh, bright, and cheery essential oils combine in this recipe to ease nausea and help the body recover from bouts of queasiness. The therapeutic effects of these oils combined can help alleviate motion and morning sickness as well. A roller bottle makes this the perfect blend when you are on the go.

2 drops ginger

2 drops lemon

2 drops peppermint

1 tablespoon carrier oil of choice

_____

½-ounce (15 ml) tinted glass
   roller bottle

3 pipettes

1 small funnel

1. Add the essential oils to the roller bottle using pipettes.

2. Using the funnel, fill the bottle with the carrier oil. Place the roller and cap on the bottle and shake well.

3. Apply a small amount to the inside of the wrists and massage it in well. While doing this, apply gentle pressure to the center of one wrist and hold it for 10 seconds. This area is a pressure point that is linked to the stomach and can help further relieve nausea. Repeat application and 10 seconds of pressure on the pressure point as needed for relief from nausea.

TIP: *For younger children, substitute spearmint for peppermint in this recipe. If you have sensitive skin, apply these oils (1 drop each) to an inhaler and inhale as needed for nausea relief.*

UPSET STOMACH AND INDIGESTION MASSAGE BLEND

Topical ✳ Safe for ages 10+

The essential oils in this blend can calm an upset stomach, as well as quiet the pain and tumult that can result from indigestion and stomach troubles. Antispasmodic oils in this blend bring serenity to a distressed stomach. The gentle, crisp blend of these aromas also promotes feelings of peace and comfort.

6 drops tangerine

4 drops spearmint

3 drops basil

3 drops ginger

2 tablespoons carrier oil
 of choice

———

1-ounce tinted glass bottle
 with lid

4 pipettes

1 small funnel

1. Add the essential oils to the bottle using pipettes.

2. Using the funnel, fill the bottle with the carrier oil. Secure the lid on the container and shake gently to blend.

3. Apply a small amount to the abdomen and massage it into the skin thoroughly. Use this blend up to three times daily for stomach issues.

TIP: *For indigestion, also try drinking a cup of peppermint, fennel, ginger, or chamomile tea. You can even combine all these dried herbs in a tea infuser to make a very effective remedy that works well alongside essential oil use.*

DIGESTION HEALTH ABDOMINAL MASSAGE BLEND

Topical ✳ *Safe for ages 10+*

Essential oils that promote digestive health and balance come together in this effective blend. This blend is perfect for those suffering from bouts of constipation, diarrhea, irritable bowel syndrome, or other conditions that affect the digestive system.

6 drops chamomile

4 drops peppermint

4 drops lemon

4 drops cardamom

4 drops ginger

2 tablespoons carrier oil of choice

———

1-ounce tinted glass bottle with lid

5 pipettes

1 small funnel

1. Add the essential oils to the bottle using pipettes.

2. Using the funnel, fill the bottle with the carrier oil. Secure the lid on the bottle and shake gently to blend.

3. Apply a small amount of this blend to the abdomen and massage it in thoroughly. If you are suffering from chronic bowel issues, do this once daily. For other issues, use as needed.

EARACHE RELIEF ROLLER BLEND

Topical ✳ *Safe for ages 10+*

This antimicrobial blend helps to combat infection and irritation in the ear. When applied to the outer ear area, it can penetrate into the tissues and help provide relief from tenderness, inflammation, and issues caused by bacteria.

3 drops tea tree

2 drops copaiba

1 drop oregano

1 tablespoon carrier oil of choice

———

½-ounce (15 ml) tinted glass
    roller bottle

1 small funnel

3 pipettes

1.   Add the essential oils to the roller bottle using pipettes.

2.   Using the funnel, fill the bottle with the carrier oil. Place the roller and cap on the bottle and shake well.

3.   Apply this blend to the outer ear only. Never use an essential oil inside the ear. Massage a small amount into the outer ear area until it is fully absorbed into the skin. Do this twice daily to help with an earache.

TIP: *There is a difference between "oil of oregano" and "oregano essential oil." Oregano essential oil is much more potent and should be used with great care. Oil of oregano is much gentler because it is made by infusing the herb into carrier oil, rather than any kind of distillation process. If you are sensitive to oregano essential oil, oil of oregano is a great alternative that presents a lower risk for skin irritation. It is also a better choice for children.*

ECZEMA EASE BLEND

Topical ✳ *Safe for ages 8+*

Antihistamine essential oils pair with anti-inflammatory and soothing oils in this blend to help manage the symptoms of eczema. Blending these oils with food-grade aloe vera gel cools the irritated area. Together, these ingredients also help relieve the itch associated with this autoimmune condition.

5 drops tea tree

5 drops lavender

4 drops rose absolute

4 drops geranium

2 tablespoons food-grade aloe
   vera gel

———

1-ounce jar with lid

4 pipettes

1. Add the essential oils to the jar.

2. Add the aloe vera gel. Using a small spoon or utensil, stir the oils and aloe vera well. Place the lid securely on the container and shake gently to blend.

3. Apply a dab of this blend to affected areas, making sure you massage it into the skin well.

4. This can be used up to three times daily to combat eczema. Store it in the fridge to keep it cool.

TIP: *Avoid scratching eczema if you can. Scratching can break open the skin, exposing it to bacteria and other pathogens, which can worsen the inflammation and cause more issues.*

FEVER REDUCTION ROLLER BLEND

Topical ✳ *Safe for ages 10+*

Peppermint is one of the most well-known essential oils for providing a cooling effect. Not only is this highly aromatic plant great for reducing fever, but it is also great for relieving pain and opening up the airways. Lemongrass essential oil has also been traditionally used for fever reduction, as well as for its antimicrobial and relaxing properties.

7 drops peppermint
7 drops lemongrass
1 tablespoon carrier oil of choice

———

½-ounce (15 ml) tinted glass
   roller bottle
2 pipettes
1 small funnel

1. Add the essential oils to the roller bottle using the pipettes.

2. Place the funnel on the bottle and fill with the carrier oil. Place the roller and cap on the bottle and shake well.

3. Apply the roller directly to the temples, back of the neck, and forehead when you are suffering from a fever. Massage the oil into the places you apply it. Be careful not to get this in your eyes.

4. Apply every 3 to 4 hours as needed for fevers.

TIP: *Taking a tepid bath can also help reduce the fever.*

HEADACHE AID ROLLER REMEDY

*Topical * Safe for ages 10+*

This combination of analgesic essential oils works synergistically to alleviate pain from headaches when they are caused by tension, stress, and related triggers.

6 drops lavender

5 drops copaiba

4 drops peppermint

4 drops birch

1 tablespoon carrier oil of choice

———

½-ounce (15 ml) tinted glass
roller bottle

1 small funnel

4 pipettes

1. Add the essential oils to the roller bottle using pipettes.

2. Using the funnel, fill the bottle with the carrier oil. Place the roller and cap on the bottle and shake well.

3. Apply a small amount of this roller remedy to the temples, or wherever you feel the most pain and pressure during a headache. Gently massage it in with your index fingers until it is fully absorbed. Be careful not to get this in your eyes.

TIP: *This remedy is most effective when used at the very onset of a headache or migraine.*

HORMONE BALANCE MASSAGE BLEND

Topical ✳ *Safe for ages 18+*

An imbalance in hormones can cause a variety of issues. Whether it is heavy or absent periods, acne, infertility, or mood swings, hormonal imbalance can wreak havoc on the body. Provide your body with hormonal balance using this powerful massage blend.

6 drops vitex

5 drops clary sage

4 drops bergamot

2 tablespoons carrier oil
   of choice

———

1-ounce tinted glass bottle
   with lid

3 pipettes

1 small funnel

1. Add the essential oils to the bottle using pipettes.

2. Using the funnel, fill the bottle with the carrier oil. Secure the lid on the bottle and shake gently to blend.

3. Massage a small amount into the lower abdomen once daily for hormone imbalance, and up to twice daily if you suffer from PCOS or absent periods.

TIP: *See a medical professional if you go several months without a menstrual period and are not going through menopause. Your body could be at risk for early menopause if you wait too long, which could result in weak or brittle bones. Vitex herb also comes in a powdered capsule form, and this can be taken internally to balance hormones.*

PMS BATH SOAK

Topical ✳ *Safe for ages 15+*

Premenstrual syndrome can cause fatigue, mood swings, headaches, and other hormonal issues. Try this recipe to help combat unwanted PMS symptoms and promote relaxation.

2 tablespoons carrier oil of choice

10 drops clary sage

8 drops ylang-ylang

8 drops jasmine

7 drops sandalwood

6 drops tangerine

1 cup Epsom salt

1. Place the carrier oil in a mixing bowl. Add the essential oils to the carrier oil and stir well.

2. Add the Epsom salt to the oils and stir thoroughly.

3. Run a warm bath and add the contents of the bowl to the bath. Soak in the bath for as long as desired. Repeat this self-care routine daily in the week prior to your menstrual cycle.

MENSTRUAL CRAMP EASE ROLLER

Topical ✳ *Safe for ages 15+*

Painful menstrual cramps don't have to be suffered through! Essential oils can relax the uterine muscles, as well as help with spasmodic pain and discomfort associated with cramping.

4 drops clary sage

4 drops chamomile

4 drops copaiba

3 drops marjoram

1 tablespoon carrier oil of choice

———

½-ounce (15 ml) tinted glass roller bottle

4 pipettes

1 small funnel

1. Add the essential oils to the roller bottle using pipettes.

2. Using the funnel, fill the bottle with the carrier oil. Place the roller and cap on the bottle and shake well.

3. Apply directly to the lower abdomen area, above the uterus, when you are experiencing cramping. Massage it thoroughly into the skin up to twice daily for relief.

TIP: *Apply a hot water bottle or heat pad to the area for further pain relief.*

FERTILITY MASSAGE BLEND

Topical ✳ *Safe for ages 18+*

Infertility is a distressing struggle for many. Essential oils that help balance hormones and increase arousal and sexual energy may help promote fertility in those seeking to conceive.

6 drops vitex

6 drops jasmine

2 tablespoons carrier oil
   of choice

———

1-ounce tinted glass bottle
   with lid

2 pipettes

1 small funnel

1. Add the essential oils to the bottle using pipettes.

2. Using the funnel, fill the bottle with the carrier oil. Secure the lid on the container and shake gently to blend.

3. Apply a small amount to the lower abdomen once daily for help with fertility. Discontinue use as soon as you become pregnant.

TIP: *Stress can negatively impact fertility, which is difficult to alleviate when you are worried about your fertility. However, do whatever you can to promote a stress-free life. Yoga, acupuncture, and regular exercise can help promote lower stress levels and possibly increase your chances of conceiving.*

CANKER SORE MOUTHWASH

Topical ✳ *Safe for ages 10+*

Canker sores can be painful. They are a type of ulcer that forms in the mouth. Trauma to the area, stress, genetic factors, allergies, and hormones can all contribute to the formation of these sores. Essential oils that kill bacteria, protect the wound, ease pain, and promote healing are great for getting rid of an unwelcome canker sore.

⅓ cup distilled water
2 drops clove
1 drop cardamom
1 drop cinnamon
1 drop thyme
2 teaspoons salt
1 teaspoon baking soda

———————

8-ounce canning jar with lid

1. Add the distilled water and essential oils to the container.

2. Add the salt and baking soda, close the lid tightly, and shake vigorously to blend the ingredients well.

3. Pour 1 or 2 tablespoons into a glass and then into your mouth.

4. Swish the liquid in your mouth for 2 to 3 minutes and then spit it out. Rinse your mouth out with plain water.

5. Repeat this up to twice daily to combat canker sores.

TOOTHACHE HELP BLEND

Topical ✳ *Safe for ages 15+*

Toothaches can be one of the most painful experiences a person can have because teeth contain nerves that can become irritated and inflamed, in addition to the surrounding tissues. Cloves have been used for centuries to alleviate the pain from a toothache. Chamomile is another analgesic and can relieve spasmodic nerve pain associated with a toothache.

2 drops chamomile

1 drop clove

1 teaspoon olive oil

———

1 small container with lid

1. Add the essential oils and olive oil to the container.

2. Close the lid tightly and shake to mix.

3. Dip your index finger in the oil blend and gently apply a small amount of the oil to the affected area. Apply up to twice daily for pain. Try to use a small amount of oil and avoid swallowing if possible.

TIP: *Ingestion of essential oils is not advised, so avoid using too much of this blend in the mouth. If you are especially sensitive to essential oils, another great option is to purchase whole cloves and chew one or hold one between the teeth on the affected area.*

RASH RELIEF ROLLER BLEND

Topical ✳ *Safe for ages 6+*

Calming essential oils work to relieve inflammation and redness, as well as promote the healing of irritated tissues. Lavender essential oil also helps with itchy skin. The antimicrobial properties of the oils in this blend will also reduce the risk of bacteria causing a skin infection. Sweet almond oil provides a thin base that will not clog pores and aggravate already irritated skin.

5 drops lavender
5 drops frankincense
1 tablespoon sweet almond oil

———————

½-ounce (15 ml) tinted glass
    roller bottle
2 pipettes
1 small funnel

1. Add the essential oils to the roller bottle using pipettes.

2. Using the funnel, fill the bottle with the sweet almond oil. Place the roller and cap on the bottle and shake well.

3. Apply this blend to your fingertips and then to the rash (don't apply from the bottle, as the rash might be contagious and contaminate the bottle). Apply up to twice daily for best results.

ANTIFUNGAL ROLLER REMEDY

Topical ✳ *Safe for ages 10+*

A powerful combination of antifungal essential oils makes this blend unstoppable when it comes to relief from fungal issues like ringworm. This blend can have you spot-free in as little as 24 hours.

10 drops lavender

10 drops tea tree

3 drops clove

1 tablespoon carrier oil of choice

———

½-ounce (15 ml) tinted glass
   roller bottle

3 pipettes

1 small funnel

1. Add the essential oils to the roller bottle using pipettes.

2. Using the funnel, fill the bottle with the carrier oil. Place the roller and cap on the bottle and shake well.

3. Apply a small amount to the affected area and cover it with a bandage. Apply and cover up to three times daily until the area is clear.

TIP: *This recipe can be modified for younger children by leaving out the clove essential oil.*

SCAR ERASER ROLLER BLEND

Topical ✳ *Safe for ages 10+*

The essential oils in this blend can help lighten scars, reduce raised spots (keloid scars), and soften the area. A synergistic blend of oils that work to tone, balance, soften, and heal skin can lead to less noticeable scarring. The castor oil in this blend also helps to heal the skin.

5 drops frankincense

3 drops cypress

3 drops geranium

3 drops neroli

3 drops sandalwood

1½ teaspoons castor oil

1½ teaspoons sweet almond or
grapeseed oil

––––––––

½-ounce (15 ml) tinted glass
roller bottle

1 small funnel

5 pipettes

1. Add the essential oils to the roller bottle using pipettes.

2. Using the funnel, fill the bottle with the carrier oils. Place the roller and cap on the bottle and shake well.

3. Apply this blend directly to scars, massaging it in well after applying. You can do this up to twice daily to help with scar healing.

SINUS PAIN AND PRESSURE ROLLER REMEDY

Topical ✳ *Safe for ages 10+*

This roller blend can be applied topically to get straight to the affected area and begin killing bacteria, opening the airways, and providing relief from pain and pressure. The naturally antibacterial, antimicrobial, analgesic, and anti-inflammatory nature of these oils can help target infection and provide relief.

6 drops tea tree

4 drops eucalyptus

4 drops peppermint

4 drops copaiba

1 tablespoon carrier oil of choice

———

½-ounce (15 ml) tinted glass
   roller bottle

4 pipettes

1 small funnel

1. Add the essential oils to the roller bottle using pipettes.

2. Using the funnel, fill the bottle with the carrier oil. Place the roller and cap on the bottle and shake well.

3. Apply this to the sinuses, focusing on the areas to the right and left of the nose, as well as the forehead. You may also want to massage it into the temples. Take extreme care not to get this in the eyes. Massage it in thoroughly to help the oils absorb into the skin and get to where they need to go to fight infection and congestion.

TIP: *In addition to using essential oils for sinus issues, try using a neti pot to further clear the sinuses.*

SINUS PAIN AND PRESSURE INHALATION REMEDY

Direct Inhalation ✳ Safe for ages 10+

Combining peppermint, clove, and oregano creates a powerful blend that clears congestion and fights infection. Together, these oils can provide relief from sinus pressure and pain.

6 drops peppermint

4 drops clove

4 drops oregano

———

1 aromatherapy inhaler

3 pipettes

Place the essential oils onto the cotton wick of the inhaler using pipettes. Snap the cap firmly into place. When you begin feeling like you have excess mucus and congestion, hold the inhaler under your nose and breathe normally for 1 to 2 minutes. Wait 10 minutes between uses and repeat this throughout the day until you begin to feel better.

TIP: *In addition to this inhalation treatment, you may also want to try a steam treatment by simply taking a hot shower or leaning over a steaming pot of water to inhale the vapor.*

INFLAMMATION BUSTER ROLLER BLEND

Topical ✳ *Safe for ages 10+*

This blend of anti-inflammatory, cooling, and healing essential oils works to reduce swelling, redness, and irritation of the skin due to trauma or inflammatory conditions like allergies.

10 drops ginger

8 drops frankincense

5 drops lemongrass

1 tablespoon carrier oil of choice

———

½-ounce (15 ml) tinted glass
  roller bottle

3 pipettes

1 small funnel

1. Add the essential oils to the roller bottle using pipettes.

2. Using the funnel, fill the bottle with the carrier oil. Place the roller and cap on the bottle and shake well.

3. Apply this to areas where the skin is inflamed and irritated, up to twice daily. Avoid areas where there is excessive trauma or open wounds.

ADULT SLEEP DIFFUSION BLEND

Diffusion ✳ *Safe for ages 15+*

Sleep provides our bodies with time to heal, repair, build the immune system, regulate hormones, and regenerate as a whole. When we are not getting enough sleep, we can suffer by being at a higher risk for contracting an illness (weakened immune system) or have trouble focusing on everyday tasks. If you are tired of lying awake at night, try diffusing this combination of grounding, calming, and gently tranquilizing essential oils.

3 drops vetiver

3 drops patchouli

2 drops valerian

———

1 ultrasonic diffuser

1. Fill the diffuser with water up to the water line. Add the essential oils to the diffuser around 30 minutes before you plan on going to bed.

2. Let it run for 10 to 15 minutes and then shut it off. If your diffuser has a timer, bring it to your room at bedtime and turn it back on as you lay in bed for another 10 to 15 minutes.

TIP: *Did you know that looking at computer and phone screens can affect your sleep? Avoid these things at least an hour prior to bedtime. Try taking a relaxing bath with Epsom salt an hour before bedtime as well.*

CHILDREN'S SLEEP REMEDY

Topical ✳ *Safe for ages 5+*

Some essential oils can be too strong for children, but the oils in this blend are gentle and effective for helping settle and soothe a restless child.

3 drops lavender

3 drops chamomile

1 tablespoon carrier oil of choice

———

½-ounce (15 ml) tinted glass roller bottle

2 pipettes

1 small funnel

1. Add the essential oils to the roller bottle using pipettes.

2. Using the funnel, fill the bottle with the carrier oil. Place the roller and cap on the bottle and shake well.

3. Apply a small amount to the chest 30 minutes prior to bedtime, preferably after bath time.

TIP: *Get a bedtime routine established early on to promote healthy sleeping habits.*

SEIZE THE DAY INHALATION BLEND

Direct Inhalation ✳ *Safe for ages 5+*

Learn to wake up without coffee using this aromatic and invigorating blend! If you are trying to kick the coffee habit, or simply have an especially hard time waking up in the morning, this is the blend for you!

---

2 drops vanilla absolute
1 drop lemon
1 drop grapefruit
1 drop orange

———

1 aromatherapy inhaler
4 pipettes

Place the essential oils onto the cotton wick of the inhaler using pipettes. Snap the cap firmly into place. Take 3 to 5 deep breaths of the inhaler upon waking in the morning.

TIP: *Avoid hitting that snooze button in the morning and try to get out of bed when your alarm goes off. Pushing the snooze button prolongs the inevitable and further encourages drowsiness.*

RESTLESS LEG SPRAY BLEND

Topical ✳ *Safe for ages 10+*

Restless legs can be quite bothersome, especially when you are trying to fall asleep. The constant urge to move the legs can prevent sleep for hours. Some describe restless leg syndrome as a crawling or tingling sensation, whereas other claim it is an aching feeling. The antispasmodic blend of essential oils in this recipe calms the urge to move the legs, in addition to easing aching and discomfort.

6 drops chamomile

5 drops petitgrain

5 drops marjoram

2 tablespoons distilled water

1-ounce tinted glass spray bottle

3 pipettes

1 small funnel

1. Add the essential oils to the spray bottle using the pipettes.

2. Using the funnel, add the distilled water to the bottle. Close the lid and shake vigorously.

3. Apply immediately after shaking the bottle by misting all over the legs. This blend works best when applied 20 minutes prior to bedtime. This also gives it time to dry.

TIP: *Avoid exercising at least an hour before bed to promote relaxation and help the body settle. Combine this recipe with the Adult Sleep Diffusion Blend (page 98) for a great night's sleep.*

SORE MUSCLES MASSAGE BLEND

Topical ✳ *Safe for ages 12+*

Stimulating and analgesic essential oils pair with healing and restoring oils in this massage blend. A carrier blend of castor and jojoba oils further ensure healing and absorption of the essential oils to help relieve pain, tension, and achiness.

5 drops chamomile
5 drops helichrysum
4 drops black pepper
4 drops wintergreen
2 drops marjoram
3 tablespoons jojoba oil
1 tablespoon castor oil

———

2-ounce tinted glass bottle
  with lid
5 pipettes
1 small funnel

1. Add the essential oils to the bottle using the pipettes.

2. Using the funnel, add the jojoba oil and castor oil to the bottle. Secure the lid on the bottle and shake gently to blend.

3. Thoroughly massage into sore muscles until it is fully absorbed, using circular motions. Use up to twice a day for best results. Avoid getting this in cuts or wounds.

SORE MUSCLES BATH SOAK

Topical ✳ *Safe for ages 12+*

The essential oils in this blend work to ease tension and relieve pain. Combining these oils with Epsom salt in a warm bath can promote healing and regeneration of tired, sore muscles.

2 tablespoons carrier oil
  of choice
15 drops lavender
15 drops helichrysum
10 drops clary sage
1 cup Epsom salt

1. Place the carrier oil in a mixing bowl. Add the essential oils to the carrier oil and stir well.

2. Add the Epsom salt to the oils and stir thoroughly.

3. Run a warm bath and add the contents of the bowl to the bath. Soak in the bath for as long as possible, making sure to fully immerse your body in the water. Do this once daily when experiencing muscles soreness and tension.

MUSCLE SPASM MASSAGE BLEND

Topical ✳ *For ages 10+*

A combination of antispasmodic, soothing, and calming essential oils make this massage blend effective for damaged muscles prone to spasms and twitching.

10 drops chamomile

8 drops clary sage

5 drops vetiver

¼ cup carrier oil of choice

———

2-ounce tinted glass bottle
with lid

3 plastic pipettes

1 small funnel

1. Add the essential oils to the bottle using pipettes.

2. Using the funnel, fill the bottle with the carrier oil. Secure the lid on the bottle and shake well.

3. Gently massage this blend into muscles prone to spasms until fully absorbed. This can be applied up to twice daily.

SPRAIN CARE MASSAGE BLEND

Topical ✳ *Safe for ages 6+*

This blend of anti-inflammatory and pain-relieving essential oils works to soothe swelling and ease pain when applied to a sprain. It can provide comfort and relief when you need it the most.

4 drops helichrysum

4 drops ginger

4 drops chamomile

4 drops peppermint

2 tablespoons carrier oil
   of choice

———

1-ounce tinted glass bottle
   with lid

4 pipettes

1 small funnel

1. Add the essential oils to the bottle using pipettes.

2. Using the funnel, fill the bottle with the carrier oil. Place the lid securely on the container and shake gently to blend.

3. To apply, dip your index finger in the oil and gently massage a small amount into the affected area, making sure to let it fully absorb into the skin.

4. Apply this massage oil up to three times daily to help manage the symptoms of a sprain. Do not get the oils in any open wounds.

TIP: *Applying ice to the area, as well as elevating the affected area, will further help with swelling and pain.*

SUNSCREEN BLEND

Topical ✳ *For ages 18+*

Some carrier oils actually offer protection from the sun's rays. Both carrot seed and raspberry seed oil can help protect the skin during times of mild to moderate sun exposure while also delivering antioxidants and beneficial omega fatty acids. Coconut oil also provides a small amount of sun protection. Helichrysum essential oil works to nourish and calm the skin.

1 cup coconut oil

2 tablespoons carrot seed oil

2 tablespoons raspberry seed oil

10 drops helichrysum

———

12-ounce container with lid

1. Blend the oils together well. You may want to melt the coconut oil to help mix the oils thoroughly.

2. Add the helichrysum and mix thoroughly.

3. Apply this blend to exposed areas of the body to protect them from the sun's rays. Apply as often as needed throughout the day. If you are prone to burning easily or are fair skinned, do not use this as your primary sunscreen. Always check your skin throughout the day to make sure you are not becoming burned. If you notice redness, stay out of the sun.

TIP: *Essential oils are great for many purposes, but no matter what people may swear by, do not use them as your only form of sun protection. The best form of sun protection is keeping the skin covered with sun-protective clothing and a wide-brimmed hat.*

SOOTHE A SUNBURN

Topical ✳ *Safe for ages 5+*

Sunburns can be painful, as well as harmful, to the skin. Help relieve the burning and soothe irritated, inflamed skin with a combination of lavender and chamomile essential oils. Aloe vera gel creates a cooling, anti-inflammatory base for this helpful recipe.

8 drops lavender

8 drops chamomile

¼ cup food-grade aloe vera gel

———

2-ounce jar with lid

1. Add the aloe vera gel to the jar.

2. Add the essential oils to the jar. Mix everything together well.

3. Apply this salve liberally to sunburned areas, up to three times daily for relief.

COOLING SPRAY FOR HOT DAYS

Topical ✻ *Safe for ages 10+ years*

If you are having a hard time cooling off on those hot, humid days, try this cooling spray to help refresh skin with a combination of enlivening oils like peppermint and lime. In addition, the aromas in this blend will instantly revive a tired body and mind!

8 drops peppermint

6 drops lime

3 tablespoons plus 1½ teaspoons distilled water

———

2-ounce tinted glass spray bottle

1 small funnel

2 pipettes

1. Place the essential oils in the bottle using pipettes.

2. Using the funnel, add the water to the bottle. Secure the sprayer on the bottle.

3. Shake the bottle well before spraying the arms, legs, chest, and back of the neck.

4. Apply up to twice daily for refreshment. Shake before each use to properly distribute the oils. Lime essential oil can be phototoxic, so avoid prolonged exposure to the sun when using this blend.

SUNBURN REMEDY SPRAY

Topical ✳ *Safe for ages 5+*

This cooling mist consists of soothing and anti-inflammatory essential oils that can help damaged skin heal, as well as relieve pain and inflammation. This easy-to-apply recipe is perfect to have on hand during the summer months!

5 drops lavender

4 drops chamomile

3 drops spearmint

2 tablespoons distilled water

———

1-ounce tinted glass spray bottle

3 pipettes

1 small funnel

1. Add the essential oils to the spray bottle using the pipettes.

2. Using the funnel, fill the bottle with the distilled water.

3. Screw the sprayer on the bottle and shake it vigorously to mix the ingredients. Because oil and water do not blend well for very long, you will need to shake this blend well before each application.

4. Lightly mist the affected areas up to three times daily.

VIRUS BUSTER DIFFUSION BLEND

Diffusion ✳ *Safe for ages 10+*

This blend of essential oils can both cleanse and purify the air in the home when a virus strikes, as well as help boost the immune system to help our bodies fight unwelcome hosts.

---

4 drops melissa

3 drops cinnamon

3 drops ravensara

3 drops clove

3 drops oregano

———

1 ultrasonic diffuser

1. Fill the diffuser with water up to the water line. Add the essential oils to the diffuser.

2. Turn on the diffuser and let it diffuse for 20 minutes. Wait an hour and repeat until the diffuser is empty. You can also move the diffuser around from room to room and let it diffuse for 20 minutes in each room.

TIP: *Choose rooms where people congregate so you can purify areas that probably contain the most pathogens.*

VIRUS BUSTER ROLLER BLEND

Topical ✳ *Safe for ages 10+*

For some viruses, it may be more effective to try a topical application of essential oils. This blend works well for viruses like shingles and herpes but can also be effective for a variety of other illnesses. Additionally, these oils can kill bacteria and provide relief from respiratory issues.

5 drops lavender

5 drops tea tree

5 drops melissa

3 drops lemon

1 tablespoon carrier oil of choice

————

½-ounce (15 ml) tinted glass roller bottle

1 small funnel

4 pipettes

1. Add the essential oils to the roller bottle using pipettes.

2. Using the funnel, fill the bottle with the carrier oil. Place the roller and cap on the bottle and shake well.

3. Apply this blend to your fingers and then to the areas affected by shingles or herpes. For all other viruses, apply to the back of the neck and pulse points such as the wrists and insides of the elbows. If applying to the wrists, bring them up to your nose and inhale deeply throughout the day.

WOUND CARE COMPRESS BLEND

*Topical * Safe for ages 10+*

This blend of skin-regenerating essential oils fights infections that make wounds red, inflamed, and sore. Do not apply this blend to serious open wounds; it is intended for mild to moderate cuts and scrapes.

6 drops lavender

6 drops tea tree

5 drops helichrysum

3 drops myrrh

1 cup distilled water

———

16-ounce canning jar with lid

1. Add the essential oils to the jar.

2. Add the distilled water, secure the lid tightly, and vigorously shake the contents.

3. Immediately place a small cloth in the container to soak up the contents. Wring the cloth out into the jar.

4. Apply the compress to the affected area up to twice daily. Use cool water to help soothe sore and inflamed tissues.

TIP: *As soon as you get a wound, clean it with soap and water to prevent infection. Keep the wound as clean as possible. Cover it and reapply a cover two to three times daily if needed to promote healing. When the wound is no longer open, you can leave it uncovered.*

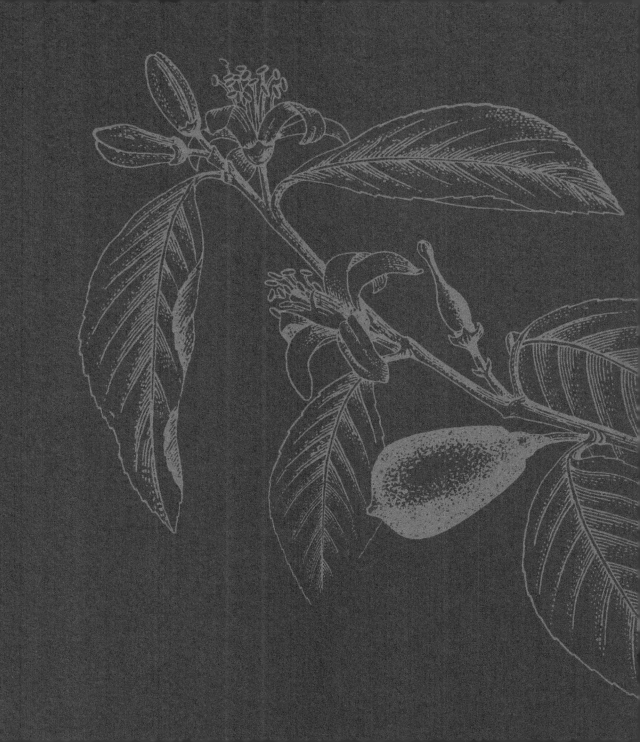

CHAPTER SIX

Emotional and Mental Well-being

Aromatherapy isn't just wonderful for the physical body; it is perfect for the mind as well. The inhalation and/or application of essential oils has been proven to help ease negative emotions and mental states while providing a sense of well-being and security. This chapter covers a wide range of uses for essential oils to foster emotional and mental well-being. You will learn how to use oils to combat panic attacks, anxiety, nervousness and frustration, depression, grief, mood swings, confusion, brain fog, mental exhaustion and fatigue, restlessness, self-confidence, anger, memory issues, distraction/focus issues, fear, stress, listlessness, apathy, burnout, stagnation, vulnerability, and pessimistic tendencies.

ANGER ALLEVIATION INHALATION BLEND

Direct Inhalation ✳ *Safe for ages 6+*

Holding on to anger can lead to anxiety, stress, apprehension, frustration, and all kinds of negative emotions. Living every day this way can wear on a body physically as well. Rose promotes a sense of comfort and encouragement, while bergamot is gently soothing and can dispel feelings of anger, frustration, and agitation. Combined, these oils can help you let go of negative and harmful emotions and find a place of rest and serenity.

3 drops rose absolute

3 drops bergamot

———

1 aromatherapy inhaler

2 pipettes

Place the essential oils onto the cotton wick of the inhaler using pipettes. Snap the cap firmly into place. Keep this blend with you at all times and take 3 to 5 deep breaths of the oils inside when you are feeling frustrated, angry, agitated, or combative. Repeat this breathing every 10 minutes as needed.

DIMINISH IRRITABILITY BATH SOAK BLEND

*Topical * Safe for ages 10+*

Irritability can be the result of a wide array of stressors. Calming and uplifting essential oils mix well in this bath soak. If you are in need of some alone time to relax and destress, this blend is perfect for you.

2 tablespoons carrier oil of choice

15 drops neroli

10 drops chamomile

10 drops sandalwood

1 to 2 cups Epsom salt

1. Place the carrier oil in a mixing bowl. Add the essential oils to the carrier oil and stir well.

2. Add the Epsom salt to the oils and stir thoroughly.

3. Run a warm bath and add the contents of the bowl to the bath. Soak for as long as you need, making sure to practice deep breathing for relaxation. Repeat this nightly, if desired.

ANXIETY INHALATION REMEDY

Direct Inhalation ✱ Safe for ages 5+

If you're prone to excessive worrying and nervousness, this remedy is for you. In this blend, a combination of nutmeg, valerian, and citronella work synergistically to promote a relaxed and calm state. Together, they relieve anxiety while gently lifting the spirits.

7 drops nutmeg

7 drops citronella

2 drops valerian

———

1 aromatherapy inhaler

3 plastic pipettes

Place the essential oils onto the cotton wick of the inhaler using the pipettes. Snap the cap firmly into place. Bring this inhaler along with you wherever you go for help with everyday anxiety, nervousness, tension, worry, and frustration. Take 3 to 5 deep breaths with your eyes closed, focusing solely on the aroma. Do this as needed for anxiety.

ANXIETY

PANIC ATTACK INHALATION REMEDY

Direct Inhalation ✻ *Safe for ages 10+*

Anxiety isn't just a problem for one's mental health. It can also manifest physical symptoms and, in some cases, panic attacks, which can involve rapid breathing and heart palpitations. This oil blend is comprised of sedative oils that provide serious calming. Together, these oils ground, soothe, and comfort during a panic attack.

10 drops melissa
6 drops vanilla absolute
3 drops valerian

1 aromatherapy inhaler
3 plastic pipettes

Place the essential oils onto the cotton wick of the inhaler using pipettes. Snap the cap firmly into place. When you feel a panic attack coming on, take out your inhaler and take 3 to 5 deep breaths with your eyes closed. Try to focus on the aroma and ground yourself. Tell yourself that you are safe. Wait a minute before taking 3 to 5 more deep breaths. Use this as needed during, or prior to, times of panic.

TIP: *Carry this inhaler with you wherever you go, as one never knows when they might experience a panic attack.*

DISPEL APATHY INHALATION BLEND

Direct Inhalation ✳ *Safe for ages 5+*

Apathy can be described as a lack of emotion, concern, interest, or feeling in general. Sometimes this is the result of being emotionally or mentally drained, and sometimes the problem goes deeper. Uplifting and joyful essential oils combine in this inhalation blend to bring feelings of intent, inspiration, and purpose. This blend is perfect for those who need a boost, both mental and emotional.

3 drops bergamot
2 drops lime

———

1 aromatherapy inhaler
2 pipettes

Place the essential oils onto the cotton wick of the inhaler using pipettes. Snap the cap firmly into place. Practice deep inhalation with the inhaler, taking 3 to 4 deep breaths at the beginning of each day. Another great time to use this blend is before starting a project.

LETHARGY AND LISTLESSNESS ROLLER REMEDY

Topical ✻ *Safe for ages 6+, Phototoxic*

While lethargy and listlessness can indicate a physical issue, it can also indicate an emotional or spiritual issue. We can become overwhelmed and crushed by the constant barrage of negativity emanating from various forms of media, as well as what is happening around us. For those needing a mental, emotional, or spiritual boost, a combination of lime and bergamot can help. Both of these essential oils uplift, dispel negativity, and boost energy.

4 drops lime

3 drops bergamot

1 tablespoon carrier oil of choice

½-ounce (15 ml) tinted glass roller bottle

1 small funnel

2 pipettes

1. Add the essential oils to the roller bottle using pipettes.

2. Using the funnel, fill the bottle with the carrier oil. Place the roller and cap on the bottle and shake well.

3. Apply to pulse points on the wrists and neck for best results. Use up to twice daily.

FINDING CONCENTRATION ROLLER REMEDY

Topical ✳ *Safe for ages 10+*

Trouble focusing can indicate a physical issue, but it can also indicate a mental or emotional issue rooted in anxiety, fear, or self-confidence. Grounding essential oils combine with cheerful and bright oils to create a blend that helps us redirect and concentrate on the task at hand. This blend is perfect for those who have been putting off that big project for fear they will be overwhelmed, or those who are seeking motivation to complete a personal mission.

3 drops cedarwood

3 drops orange

2 drops vetiver

1 drop ylang-ylang

1 tablespoon carrier oil of choice

———

½-ounce (15 ml) tinted glass
    roller bottle

4 pipettes

1 small funnel

1. Add the essential oils to the roller bottle using pipettes.

2. Using the funnel, fill the bottle with the carrier oil. Place the roller and cap on the bottle and shake well.

3. Apply this blend to pulse points on the wrists and neck for best results. Use up to twice daily.

TIP: *When applying a blend to pulse points on the wrists, you can further benefit from the therapeutic oils by bringing your wrists up to your nose and deeply inhaling throughout the day.*

BRAIN FOG DIFFUSION BLEND

Diffusion ✳ Safe for ages 10+

Have you ever felt like your brain was in a fog? This can be the result of too much mental pressure, stress, hormonal changes, or a lack of proper rest. There are also physical issues that could contribute to brain fog, such as liver disease and high blood pressure. This blend helps to fortify and support our mental state by providing calm and quiet to an overstressed mind. The citrus oils provide an invigorating and refreshing boost to the mind, while cedarwood promotes peace and tranquility.

4 drops cedarwood

3 drops vetiver

3 drops orange

2 drops grapefruit

———

1 ultrasonic diffuser

1. Fill the diffuser with water up to the water line. Add the essential oils to the diffuser.

2. Turn on and let the diffuser run for 20 minutes. Diffuse any time you wish to clear your head.

TIP: *A great time to diffuse this blend is during meditation, yoga, or prayer. It can be diffused prior to studying for an exam as well.*

BURNOUT DIFFUSION REMEDY

Diffusion ✳ *Safe for ages 5+*

Prolonged and repeated stress or anxiety can leave you feeling serious burnout. Those who are sick of their job due to constant stress are especially susceptible, but we can experience burnout in many other facets of life. Two of the most calming oils on the market work together in this diffusion blend to help you cope with burnout. Both lavender and sandalwood provide relief from stress and anxiety while promoting a sense of purpose and motivation.

5 drops lavender

4 drops sandalwood

———

1 ultrasonic diffuser

1. Fill the diffuser with water up to the water line. Add the essential oils to the diffuser.

2. Turn on and let the diffuser run for 20 minutes and then shut it off for at least 2 hours before repeating (only if needed).

TIP: *Diffuse this blend before and after work, or before taking on a task you are exhausted with.*

COPE WITH CHANGE DIFFUSION BLEND

Diffusion ✳ *Safe for ages 10+*

Many people have a hard time adapting to change, especially when it is sudden or unexpected. The supportive and grounding essential oils in this blend help encourage feelings of inner peace, no matter what may be changing around you. In times of instability, this blend can foster a sense of solidity on what may feel like shaky ground.

4 drops clary sage

3 drops orange

2 drops cypress

———

1 ultrasonic diffuser

1. Fill the diffuser with water up to the water line. Add the essential oils to the diffuser.

2. Turn on and let the diffuser run for 20 minutes and then shut it off for at least 2 hours before repeating (only if needed).

TIP: *Diffuse this blend on moving day, when you are switching jobs/careers, or any other times of great life change.*

TRANSITION EASE DIFFUSION BLEND

Diffusion ✳ Safe for ages 8+

Life is full of transitions! Major shifts may feel overwhelming at times, and aromatherapy can provide a sense of constancy and steadiness throughout these processes. Cypress helps you find spiritual and emotional stability, as well as strength. Bergamot is wonderful for contributing feelings of refreshment and helping to let go of negative emotions. Together, they create a blend perfect for times of transition.

5 drops cypress
5 drops bergamot

———

1 ultrasonic diffuser

1. Fill the diffuser with water up to the water line. Add the essential oils to the diffuser.

2. Turn on and let the diffuser run for 20 minutes and then shut it off for at least 2 hours before repeating (only if needed).

HUG-IN-A-BOTTLE INHALATION BLEND

Direct Inhalation ✻ *Safe for ages 6+*

The warm and comforting combination of cinnamon and vanilla evoke feelings of security and contentment. This inhalation blend promotes mental and emotional well-being in times of turmoil.

3 drops vanilla absolute

2 drops cinnamon

———

1 aromatherapy inhaler

2 pipettes

Place the essential oils onto the cotton wick of the inhaler using pipettes. Snap the cap firmly into place and bring this with you wherever you go. To use, take 4 to 6 deep breaths of the inhaler. Use as needed when you feel like you need a mental or emotional "hug."

BRING ON THE PEACE DIFFUSION BLEND

Diffusion ✳ *Safe for ages 6+*

Blissful citrus aromas pair with grounding earthy aromas in this blend to help promote peace and tranquility. This blend is perfect for those in need of relaxation and centeredness.

4 drops grapefruit

4 drops lemon

3 drops sandalwood

———

1 ultrasonic diffuser

1. Fill the diffuser with water up to the water line. Add the essential oils to the diffuser.

2. Turn on and let the diffuser run for 20 minutes and then shut it off for at least 2 hours before repeating (only if needed).

CONFUSION TO CLARITY INHALATION BLEND

Direct Inhalation ✳ *Safe for ages 10+*

Sometimes our minds can become so full of life's stresses that we become confused by things that normally wouldn't confuse us. Other times confusion is brought on by a decision that must be made and the uncertainty that comes along with it. The combination of oils in this blend bring grounding, clarity, and peace. They work together to promote a sense of stability and fortify the mind.

4 drops frankincense

4 drops vetiver

3 drops cajeput

3 drops lemongrass

2 drops rosemary

_____

1 aromatherapy inhaler

5 pipettes

Place the essential oils onto the cotton wick of the inhaler using pipettes. Snap the cap firmly into place. Carry this inhaler blend around with you throughout the day, and when you become overwhelmed with confusion and need clarity or grounding, inhale it deeply for 1 minute. Focus on the grounding and uplifting aromas and do not let your mind wander. Inhale as often as needed.

TAKE COURAGE INHALATION BLEND

Direct Inhalation ✳ *Safe for ages 6+*

This blend cultivates feelings of strength, courage, and perseverance in the midst of a tumultuous or uncertain situation. These fortifying essential oils can dissolve fear and anxiety, helping you to take hold of courage.

2 drops nutmeg

1 drop lavender

1 drop cardamom

———

1 aromatherapy inhaler

3 pipettes

Place the essential oils onto the cotton wick of the inhaler using pipettes. Snap the cap firmly into place. Deeply inhale, taking 3 to 4 breaths, when you are feeling a lack of courage. Use as needed and take with you on the go for moments you need help overcoming the fear to take on an issue.

VULNERABILITY DIFFUSION BLEND

Diffusion ✳ *Safe for ages 6+*

Nurturing essential oils combine in this diffusion blend to help provide you with the courage to open up. These oils can help ease anxiety and insecurity as well, helping you get past what is holding you back and reveal who you really are to those you love.

3 drops melissa
3 drops sandalwood

―――――

1 ultrasonic diffuser

1. Fill the diffuser with water up to the water line. Add the essential oils to the diffuser.

2. Turn on and let the diffuser run for 20 minutes and then shut it off for at least 2 hours before repeating (only if needed).

CALM CHILD ROLLER BLEND

Topical * Safe for ages 6+, Phototoxic

Sometimes children may find it hard to pay attention, becoming easily distracted, unfocused, and overstimulated. This can be the result of life changes or transitions, trauma, diet, or a wide array of triggers. In this blend, a simple combination of two soothing and grounding essential oils can help promote focus, peace, and serenity in children who are having a hard time getting settled.

5 drops vetiver

5 drops bergamot

1 tablespoon carrier oil of choice

––––––––

½-ounce (15 ml) tinted glass
    roller bottle

2 pipettes

1 small funnel

1. Add the essential oils to the roller bottle using pipettes.

2. Using the funnel, fill the bottle with the carrier oil. Place the roller and cap on the bottle and shake well.

3. Apply a small amount to the back of the neck and behind the ears up to twice daily.

EMOTIONAL AND MENTAL EXHAUSTION INHALATION BLEND

Direct Inhalation ✳ *Safe for ages 10+*

The mind and emotions can become exhausted when one is experiencing a significant amount of stress, pressure, or turmoil. Symptoms of mental or emotional exhaustion include trouble falling or staying asleep, weight loss or gain, difficulty paying attention, mood swings, irritability, frustration, anxiety, or low emotional reactions due to burnout. A blend of relaxing, soothing, and motivating essential oils helps to bring the mind to a place of rest, while promoting cheer and a sense of reassurance.

3 drops jasmine

2 drops vanilla absolute

1 drop peppermint

———

1 aromatherapy inhaler

3 plastic pipettes

Place the essential oils onto the cotton wick of the inhaler using pipettes. Snap the cap firmly into place. Take 3 to 4 deep breaths with your eyes closed, trying to focus on nothing else but the nourishing aromas. Repeat this action every 15 minutes as needed.

TIP: *Bring this blend with you on the go for times when you are feeling low or in need of an encouraging mental or emotional boost.*

DISPEL FEAR ROLLER BLEND

*Topical * Safe for ages 6+, Phototoxic*

If you are seeking help for worry and fear, this blend is perfect for you. If you feel like constant fears are preventing you from fully experiencing life, these elevating oils can dispel the fear and replace it with peace, joy, and tranquility.

6 drops bergamot

3 drops neroli

2 drops frankincense

1 tablespoon carrier oil of choice

———

½-ounce (15 ml) tinted glass roller bottle

3 pipettes

1 small funnel

1. Add the essential oils to the roller bottle using the pipettes.

2. Using the funnel, fill the bottle with the carrier oil. Place the roller and cap on the bottle and shake well.

3. Apply to pulse points on the wrists and neck for best results. Use up to twice daily.

FIND FORGIVENESS DIFFUSION BLEND

Diffusion ✳ *Safe for ages 8+*

This blend of gentle releasing and stirring essential oils helps one look inward and open their heart to either receive forgiveness or forgive themselves. If there is something you have been holding on to, this blend can help you find the strength to finally forgive, accept forgiveness, and release negative emotions.

6 drops myrrh

5 drops orange

———

1 ultrasonic diffuser

1. Fill the diffuser with water up to the water line. Add the essential oils to the diffuser.

2. Let the diffuser run for 20 minutes and then shut it off for at least 2 hours before repeating (only if needed).

GRIEF AND LOSS DIFFUSION BLEND

Diffusion ✳ Safe for ages 10+

Feelings of grief can almost overwhelm a person. These two uplifting oils combine perfectly in a diffuser during times of grief to help promote feelings of emotional well-being, easing tension, anxiety, and frayed nerves.

5 drops melissa

5 drops bergamot

———

1 ultrasonic diffuser

1. Fill the diffuser with water up to the water line. Add the essential oils to the diffuser.

2. Turn on and run the diffuser for 10 to 15 minutes and shut it off. Wait 1 or 2 hours before repeating this. Repeat as needed during times of grief and loss.

TIP: *You may also choose to run this before bedtime to help fall asleep when emotions are overwhelming you.*

HOPE RESTORATION DIFFUSION BLEND

Diffusion ✳ *Safe for ages 8+*

Feelings of hopelessness can be discouraging and lead to depression. Essential oils, along with positive affirmations and habits, can reduce these feelings and promote optimism. Citrus essential oils are naturally uplifting and can promote feelings of optimism and hope when you are feeling down. Oils like tea tree and citronella are also beneficial for clearing negativity and lack of enthusiasm for life.

3 drops lemon

3 drops orange

2 drops citronella

2 drops tea tree

1 ultrasonic diffuser

1. Fill the diffuser with water up to the water line. Add the essential oils to the diffuser.

2. Turn on and let the diffuser run for 20 minutes and shut it off. Wait an hour before turning it on again. Repeat until the water is gone.

TIP: *Combine your essential oil use with positive affirmations throughout the day to further promote positivity and cheer.*

INSPIRATION FOR A TIRED MIND DIFFUSION BLEND

Diffusion ✳ Safe for ages 6+

Cardamom not only helps to improve concentration, but it can also energize a tired mind! Tangerine elicits feelings of alertness and attentiveness, giving you motivation and inspiration to succeed in any endeavor.

5 drops cardamom

3 drops tangerine

———

1 ultrasonic diffuser

1. Fill the diffuser with water up to the water line. Add the essential oils to the diffuser.

2. Turn on and let the diffuser run for 20 minutes and then shut it off for at least 2 hours before repeating (only if needed).

TIP: *Diffuse this blend while sitting down to write your next inspiring piece, or while creating your next artistic masterpiece.*

AN INHALATION BLEND FOR LONELINESS

Direct Inhalation ❋ *Safe for ages 10+*

It is important to remember that time alone can be good for us. It can give us perspective and help us to be more comfortable with ourselves by building confidence in our own abilities. However, it's also natural to have feelings of loneliness. This blend can help quiet negative emotions during times when you feel lost or abandoned in a sea of confusion. This combination also works to lift the spirits and improve overall emotional clarity.

2 drops clary sage

2 drops rose absolute

1 drop helichrysum

——————

1 aromatherapy inhaler

3 pipettes

Place the essential oils onto the cotton wick of the inhaler using pipettes. Snap the cap firmly into place and bring this with you wherever you go. Deeply inhale, taking 3 to 4 breaths, when feelings of loneliness begin to distract you from living your best life.

LOVE ON THE MIND ROLLER BLEND

Topical ✳ Safe for ages 10+, Phototoxic

Attract what you desire with this erotic and invigorating blend of spicy, floral, and citrus essential oils. This blend is perfect for everyday application, first dates, or special moments with the one you love.

10 drops vanilla absolute

5 drops rose absolute

3 drops grapefruit

14 ml carrier oil of choice

———————

½-ounce (15 ml) tinted glass
   roller bottle

3 pipettes

1 small funnel

1. Add the essential oils to the roller bottle using pipettes.

2. Using the funnel, fill the bottle with the carrier oil. Place the roller and cap on the bottle and shake well.

3. Apply a small amount directly to pulse points like the wrists, neck, and insides of elbows. Use daily or as desired.

SENSUAL ENERGY MASSAGE BLEND

Topical ❋ Safe for ages 10+

This warming blend combines sweet and spicy for the ultimate massage experience. The skin-soothing and toning properties of rose are a treat to the skin. Black pepper provides a gentle warming sensation that helps promote circulation.

2 tablespoons carrier oil of choice

10 drops rose absolute

6 drops black pepper

———

1-ounce tinted glass bottle with lid

2 pipettes

1 small funnel

1. Add the essential oils to the carrier oil using pipettes.

2. Using the funnel, fill the bottle with the carrier oil. Secure the lid on the bottle and shake gently to blend.

3. Massage into the shoulders, back, arms, legs, and torso for a relaxing yet stimulating experience. Avoid contact with the eyes or mucous membranes.

ENHANCED MEMORY INHALATION BLEND

Direct Inhalation ✳ *Safe for ages 10+*

This combination of oils has been proven to strengthen memory, keeping you on track and focused so you are able to tackle anything the day throws at you!

4 drops rosemary

3 drops cardamom

———

1 aromatherapy inhaler

4 pipettes

Place the essential oils onto the cotton wick of the inhaler using pipettes. Snap the cap firmly into place. This blend makes a great brain stimulator when used upon waking to start your day. Simply take 3 to 5 deep breaths in the morning. You can use this throughout the day as well, up to five times daily.

TIP: *The more consistently you use this blend, the better your chances of improving memory and brain health.*

CLEAR YOUR HEAD DIFFUSION REMEDY

Diffusion ✳ *Safe for ages 10+*

Do you feel like you cannot focus due to stress? Are you feeling confused or overwhelmed? This blend is perfect for these situations and can help you focus, as well as achieve stability to see through the cloudiness.

5 drops frankincense

3 drops eucalyptus

———

1 ultrasonic diffuser

1. Fill the diffuser with water up to the water line. Add the essential oils to the diffuser.

2. Turn on and let the diffuser run for 20 minutes and then shut it off for at least 2 hours before repeating (only if needed).

MOOD SWING MANAGEMENT ROLLER BLEND

Topical ✼ *Safe for ages 10+*

This blend is for those who find they are not feeling like themselves due to mood swings associated with PMS or emotional issues. The oils in this roller blend calm, stabilize, and promote uplifting feelings of optimism in the midst of tumult.

7 drops melissa

6 drops chamomile

6 drops neroli

1 tablespoon carrier oil of choice

————

½-ounce (15 ml) tinted glass
   roller bottle

3 pipettes

1 small funnel

1. Add the essential oils to the roller bottle using pipettes.

2. Using the funnel, fill the bottle with the carrier oil. Place the roller and cap on the bottle and shake well.

3. Apply this to pulse points like the inside of the elbow, wrists, and neck when you feel like you need grounding and stabilization due to mood swings. Use as needed, up to three times daily.

EASING NERVES INHALATION BLEND

Direct Inhalation ✳ *Safe for ages 5+*

When you're worrying about something, it's easy for the mind to become overwhelmed with dread. Everyday tasks that normally aren't difficult can suddenly cause severe frustration. This blend contains gently sedative and uplifting oils to create feelings of peace and emotional well-being.

7 drops neroli

6 drops bergamot

5 drops sandalwood

3 drops rose absolute

_____

1 aromatherapy inhaler

4 plastic pipettes

Place the essential oils onto the cotton wick of the inhaler using the pipettes. Snap the cap firmly into place. During times when you are experiencing nervousness or frustration, deeply inhale the contents of the inhaler. Take 3 to 5 breaths with your eyes closed, focusing on the powerful aromas. Repeat as often as necessary.

NERVOUS EXHAUSTION BATH REMEDY

Topical ✳ Safe for ages 10+

Nervous exhaustion is the result of stress and anxiety. When a person has to deal with stress over and over for an extended amount of time, they may experience extreme mental, physical, and emotional fatigue. This blend of oils helps restore the body, mind, and emotions. Ravensara can help ease the mind, while lemongrass uplifts. Vetiver grounds and calms, bringing peace and comfort to anyone in need of a break.

2 tablespoons carrier oil
  of choice
15 drops lemongrass
10 drops vetiver
5 drops ravensara
1 to 2 cups Epsom salt

1. Place the carrier oil in a mixing bowl. Add the essential oils to the carrier oil and stir well.

2. Add the Epsom salt to the oils and stir thoroughly.

3. Run a warm bath and add the contents of the bowl to the bath. Soak for as long as you need, making sure to practice deep breathing for relaxation. Repeat this nightly, if desired.

INNER PATIENCE INHALATION REMEDY

Direct Inhalation ✳ *Safe for ages 6+*

Dealing with everyday stress can be hard. This blend promotes feelings of positivity and centeredness and is perfect for those seeking to improve their patience levels. Citrus, earthy, and floral aromas combine in this special blend.

3 drops neroli

2 drops bergamot

1 drop vetiver

1 drop geranium

———

1 aromatherapy inhaler

4 pipettes

Place the essential oils onto the cotton wick of the inhaler using pipettes. Snap the cap firmly into place. Deeply inhale, taking 3 to 4 breaths, when you need more patience.

TIP: *Take this inhaler blend along with you when you know you will be headed somewhere waiting is inevitable!*

NO NEGATIVITY DIFFUSION BLEND

Diffusion ✳ *Safe for ages 6+*

This blend employs essential oils that drive away negative feelings and focus on our inward person. Taking the time to meditate on your mental and emotional tendencies is vital to understanding why you are feeling a certain way. These oils can help you with this process.

5 drops cedarwood

3 drops rose absolute

3 drops cypress

———

1 ultrasonic diffuser

1. Fill the diffuser with water up to the water line. Add the essential oils to the diffuser.

2. Turn on and let the diffuser run for 10 to 20 minutes and then shut it off. During this time, meditate on your feelings and emotions and why you may be feeling negative. Inhale the aromas deeply. Repeat this every 2 to 3 hours throughout the day if needed.

SADNESS AND DEPRESSION ROLLER BLEND

Topical ✳ *Safe for ages 10+, Phototoxic*

Sadness and depression can be brought on by traumatic life events or nothing at all. Sadness can be described as feelings of sorrow, disappointment, melancholy, or despair; depression is a mood disorder characterized by constant feelings of sadness. Those with depression may lose interest in things they once enjoyed, sleep more than normal, feel lethargic, or experience feelings of hopelessness. If left untreated, depression can become serious. It is always important to seek professional help if you think you may have depression. This oil combination for topical application combines oils that calm and uplift, providing a warm and soothing feeling. They also ground the mind and provide a sense of peace.

5 drops orange

5 drops vanilla absolute

5 drops lavender

5 drops cinnamon

1 tablespoon carrier oil of choice

_____

½-ounce (15 ml) tinted glass
   roller bottle

4 pipettes

1 small funnel

1. Add the essential oils to the roller bottle using pipettes.

2. Using the funnel, fill the bottle with the carrier oil. Place the roller and cap on the bottle and shake well.

3. Apply this oil to pulse points on the neck, chest, wrist, and inner elbow up to twice daily for feelings of sadness and mild to moderate depression.

SELF-CONFIDENCE INHALATION BLEND

Direct Inhalation ✳ *Safe for ages 5+*

This combination of essential oils helps you focus and look inward. When you are able to focus on who you really are, as well as seek your true identity, you will begin to realize that there is more to life than seeking to fit into the deceptive mold society has formed for you.

2 drops clove

1 drop pine

1 drop frankincense

1 drop black pepper

———

1 aromatherapy inhaler

4 pipettes

Place the essential oils onto the cotton wick of the inhaler using pipettes. Snap the cap firmly into place and bring this with you wherever you go. To use, deeply inhale the inhaler, taking 3 to 4 hearty breaths of the aromas as needed to build self-confidence.

EMPOWERING ROLLER BLEND

Topical ✳ Safe for ages 15+

This remedy combines floral scents that can promote emotional support, self-confidence, empowerment, and sensuality. Jojoba essential oil is a great carrier oil for this blend because it is light yet nourishing to the skin.

5 drops jasmine

4 drops rose absolute

3 drops ylang-ylang

1 tablespoon jojoba oil

———

½-ounce (15 ml) tinted glass roller bottle

3 pipettes

1 small funnel

1. Add the essential oils to the roller bottle using pipettes.

2. Using the funnel, fill the bottle with the jojoba oil. Place the roller and cap on the bottle and shake well.

3. Apply a small amount to pulse points on the neck, wrists, and insides of the elbows as needed for a boost in confidence.

INHALATION BLEND FOR SHOCK AND TRAUMA

Direct Inhalation ✳ *Safe for ages 6+*

Shock and trauma occur when an adverse and unexpected event takes place in someone's life. A strong need for strength, courage, peace, and groundedness is experienced. Melissa provides comfort during times of trauma and sadness. Neroli nurtures and supports a broken spirit when you need it most.

———————————————

3 drops neroli

1 drop melissa

———

1 aromatherapy inhaler

2 pipettes

Place the essential oils onto the cotton wick of the inhaler using pipettes. Snap the cap firmly into place. Deeply inhale, taking 3 to 4 breaths every 20 minutes when you are experiencing shock or trauma.

STAGNATION

SAY GOODBYE TO STAGNATION
INHALATION BLEND

Direct Inhalation ✷ *Safe for ages 6+*

Have you ever felt like you were stuck in the same place, emotionally and mentally? Perhaps you have felt like you were not growing as you should or that you fail to take any risks necessary to evolve. Essential oils that inspire growth and progress, both mentally and emotionally, make up this lovely blend. Gentle citrus aromas combine with stimulating peppermint to create a unique and inspiring blend.

2 drops bergamot
1 drop lemongrass
1 drop peppermint

―――――
1 aromatherapy inhaler
3 pipettes

Place the essential oils onto the cotton wick of the inhaler using pipettes. Snap the cap firmly into place. To use, deeply inhale, taking 3 to 4 breaths, when you are feeling a lack of inspiration and need to overcome stagnation. Repeat as needed daily.

LONG DAY BATH SOAK FOR STRESS AND TENSION RELIEF

*Topical * Safe for ages 10+*

A combination of uplifting and tension-reducing essential oils help the body, as well as the mind, unwind. When used in a bath soak with Epsom salt, this recipe promotes muscle relaxation, stress reduction, and optimism. Look forward to tackling tomorrow with this blend!

2 tablespoons carrier oil
  of choice
15 drops chamomile
15 drops lavender
10 drops tangerine
8 drops melissa
1 to 2 cups Epsom salt

1. Place the carrier oil in a mixing bowl. Add the essential oils to the carrier oil and stir well.

2. Add the Epsom salt to the oils and stir thoroughly.

3. Run a warm bath and add the contents of the bowl to the bath. Soak for as long as you need, making sure to practice deep breathing for relaxation.

TIP: *Skip the candles during your bath and opt instead for relaxing music and dimmed lighting. Candles may be relaxing to watch, but they emit smoke and other undesirable fumes into the air.*

TENSION FROM STRESS MASSAGE BLEND

Topical ✳ *Safe for ages 12+*

Stress can do a lot of damage in a body, and tension is just one way it manifests. When you are constantly overcome with stress, anxiety, and nervousness, your body may tense up for long periods without you even realizing you are doing it. Symptoms include sore muscles in areas where the body carries tension, like the shoulders. This blend combines massage with oils that have proven tension-melting properties. It can even work to get to the root of the problem and help reduce stress in general.

10 drops frankincense

8 drops lavender

8 drops clary sage

2 tablespoons carrier oil
   of choice

———

1-ounce tinted glass bottle
   with lid

3 pipettes

1 small funnel

1. Add the essential oils to the container using pipettes.

2. Using the funnel, fill the bottle with the carrier oil. Secure the lid on the bottle and shake gently to blend.

3. This massage blend works great when applied to the shoulders, or any other areas where the body may be carrying tension from stress. Massage deeply into the skin, making sure it fully absorbs. Do this daily for relief from stress-induced tension and discomfort.

CHAPTER SEVEN

Cosmetics and Personal Care

Many cosmetics and personal care items contain ingredients like parabens, sodium lauryl sulfate (SLS), and ammonium lauryl sulfate (ALS) that can actually damage our bodies and sabotage our efforts to look and feel our best. Essential oils can replace a great number of everyday skin and hair care items, as well as provide deep nourishment. In this chapter, you will learn how to create your own natural cosmetics and personal care products to treat acne, aging skin, scars and stretch marks, cellulite, and a dull complexion. In addition, you will learn how to create your own all-natural personal care items such as soaps, shampoos, toners, deodorant, lip balm, sugar scrub, makeup remover, facial masks, steams, and even toothpaste!

ACNE FACE WASH REMEDY

Topical ✳ *Safe for ages 10+*

This antimicrobial blend treats acne in a gentle way by ridding the skin of bacteria, as well as soothing redness and inflammation. Castor oil makes a great addition as a carrier oil for this blend because it is soothing and nourishing to the skin. However, a little of this sticky oil can go a long way, so here it is mixed with sweet almond oil.

20 drops tea tree

20 drops lavender

10 drops lime

2 tablespoons castor oil

2 tablespoons sweet almond oil

———

3 pipettes

2-ounce tinted glass
  dropper bottle

1 small funnel

1. Add the essential oils to the bottle using pipettes.

2. Using the funnel, pour the castor oil into the bottle and then fill it up the rest of the way with sweet almond oil, leaving a little room at the top for the dropper to be inserted. Screw on the dropper securely and shake the mixture well.

3. Once a day, apply one dropper full of this blend to the face and leave it on for 15 minutes before washing it off.

TIP: *The shower is the perfect place to use this remedy because the steam opens the pores and lets the treatment penetrate. Avoid getting this in your eyes.*

ACNE SPOT TREATMENT BLEND

Topical ✳ *Safe for ages 10+, Phototoxic*

For more stubborn acne, a spot treatment may kill the bacteria festering inside of a pimple. Grapeseed oil is a great carrier for this spot treatment because it is lightweight, absorbs into the skin easily, and won't clog pores.

15 drops tea tree

8 drops lemon

5 drops rosemary

1 tablespoon grapeseed oil

_____

½-ounce (15 ml) tinted glass roller bottle

3 plastic pipettes

1 small funnel

1. Add the essential oils to the roller bottle using pipettes.

2. Using the funnel, fill the bottle with the grapeseed oil. Place the roller and cap on the bottle and shake well.

3. This blend works well when applied at the earliest onset of a pimple, blackhead, or whitehead. Treat up to twice a day. Use caution when applying essential oils to your face and avoid getting them in your eyes.

TIP: *Do a spot test beforehand to make sure you are not allergic.*

ACNE SCAR AWAY TREATMENT

Topical ✳ *Safe for ages 10+*

These antioxidant oils combine antiseptic properties with skin-soothing and tightening properties to relieve discoloration, fade scarring, and nourish the affected area. Jojoba oil makes a fine carrier oil for a scar blend due to its emollient properties.

15 drops frankincense

10 drops cypress

4 drops ravensara

1 tablespoon jojoba oil

———

½-ounce (15 ml) tinted glass roller bottle

3 pipettes

1 small funnel

1. Add the essential oils to the roller bottle using pipettes.

2. Using the funnel, fill the bottle with the jojoba oil. Place the roller and cap on the bottle and shake well.

3. Apply a small amount of this treatment directly to the affected area, once daily. Avoid getting it in the eyes.

FACIAL STEAM FOR HEALTHY SKIN

Diffusion ✳ *Safe for ages 15+*

Because steam can open pores and loosen blackhead-causing debris, it can promote a healthier, acne-free complexion! Not only is a facial stream treatment great for acne, but it can promote skin health and circulation. The addition of skin-regenerating essential oils gives open pores a deeply restorative treatment.

5 drops geranium

4 drops rose absolute

4 drops patchouli

―――――

Small pot

Bath towel

1. Bring a small pot of water to a boil on the stove and then turn off the heat.

2. Move the pot to another heat-safe area where you can put your face over it safely. Add the essential oils.

3. Place your face over the pot of steaming water and put a towel over your head to trap in the steam. Keep your head at least a foot away from the pot of water at all times.

4. Keep your face over the steam for 5 to 10 minutes. Repeat once weekly for healthy skin.

WRINKLE REDUCTION FACIAL TONER SPRAY

Topical ✳ *Safe for ages 10+*

Aging skin in need of tone and balance can greatly benefit from this recipe. This combination of deeply repairing and restorative essential oils hydrates skin while providing balance.

3 drops patchouli

3 drops geranium

2 drops jasmine

2 tablespoons distilled water

1 tablespoon witch hazel

1½ teaspoons vegetable glycerin

———————

2-ounce tinted glass spray bottle

1 small funnel

3 plastic pipettes

1. Add the essential oils to the bottle using pipettes.

2. Using the funnel, add the distilled water, witch hazel, and vegetable glycerin to the bottle.

3. Secure the sprayer on the bottle and shake vigorously to blend. Immediately apply 2 or 3 sprays of toner to the face after shaking. Shake before each use and use once daily for best results.

WRINKLE REDUCTION FACIAL SERUM

Topical ✳ *Safe for ages 10+*

Anti-inflammatory oils work with antioxidant oils in this serum to help regenerate and restore aging skin. Avocado oil is the perfect carrier oil for an aging skin blend because it can actually boost collagen production!

12 drops frankincense

6 drops geranium

5 drops neroli

1 tablespoon avocado oil

———

½-ounce (15 ml) tinted glass
   roller bottle

3 pipettes

1 small funnel

1. Add the essential oils to the roller bottle using pipettes.

2. Using a funnel, fill the bottle with the avocado oil. Place the roller and cap on the bottle and shake well.

3. Apply this serum directly to problem areas and areas prone to wrinkles. It is best to apply it once daily, at bedtime.

SOOTHING AND TIGHTENING EYE TREATMENT

Topical ✳ *Safe for ages 15+*

This gentle formula contains oils that can heal skin around the eyes, as well as reduce inflammation and provide elasticity. They work synergistically to restore a more youthful appearance.

10 drops helichrysum

10 drops lavender

1 tablespoon rose hip oil

⸻

½-ounce (15 ml) tinted glass
   roller bottle

2 pipettes

1 small funnel

1. Add the essential oils to the roller bottle using pipettes.

2. Using the funnel, fill the bottle with rose hip oil, leaving room to place the roller back on. Place the roller and cap on the bottle and shake well.

3. Apply a small amount of this treatment to your index finger and gently dab around the eye area in the evenings before bed. Take care not to get any in the eyes.

WRINKLE REDUCTION CLAY MASK

Topical ✳ Safe for ages 18+

For aging or dry skin, a mask with restorative and hydrating essential oils helps to nourish and protect the skin. Frankincense and clary sage are both wonderful for aging skin and reducing wrinkles and fine lines.

2 tablespoons bentonite clay

1 to 2 tablespoons water

2 drops frankincense

2 drops clary sage

1. Place the bentonite clay in a small bowl. Slowly add the water, starting with only 1 tablespoon and stirring well. Keep adding a few drops of water, up to 1 tablespoon more, until a paste-like consistency is achieved.

2. Add the essential oils and stir everything well.

3. Apply evenly to the face and leave on for 5 to 10 minutes. Rinse off gently with warm water. Repeat up to three times weekly if desired. Avoid getting this mask in the eyes.

SKIN SOFTENING SUGAR SCRUB

Topical ✳ *Safe for ages 12+*

Sugar scrubs are an amazing way to treat your body. They can help gently exfoliate and remove dead skin cells while treating the skin with therapeutic oils that bring nourishment and softness. Essential oils that calm and uplift combine in this recipe to create an invigorating, yet peaceful blend to help smooth the skin. This sugar scrub will leave your skin feeling baby-soft.

2 tablespoons shea butter

1½ tablespoons jojoba oil

1½ teaspoons castor oil

15 drops lavender

10 drops tangerine

¼ cup granulated sugar

———

8-ounce container with lid

1. Add the shea butter, jojoba oil, castor oil, and essential oils to the container and stir well.

2. Add the sugar and stir again, making sure to mix the ingredients thoroughly.

3. In the shower, gently massage the scrub into damp skin and rinse it off well.

4. Do this weekly to promote healthy, supple skin.

INVIGORATING MORNING BODY SCRUB

Topical ✻ *Safe for ages 10+*

A gently invigorating blend of peppermint and vanilla make this sugar scrub perfect for use in your morning shower or to cool off after a day's work in the sun! Peppermint wakes up the body and mind while vanilla soothes and uplifts. This recipe creates a cooling sensation on the skin that brings refreshment and rejuvenation to the body.

---

2 to 3 tablespoons carrier oil
   of choice

3 drops peppermint

3 drops vanilla absolute

½ cup granulated sugar

———

8-ounce container with lid

1. Add the carrier oil and essential oils to the container.

2. Add the sugar and stir until everything is well-blended.

3. In the shower, gently massage the scrub into damp skin and rinse it off well.

4. Repeat weekly, as desired.

LUSCIOUS SHEA BUTTER WHIPPED LOTION RECIPE

Topical ✱ *Safe for ages 10+*

Most commercial lotions contain hormone disrupters, as well as dangerous parabens and synthetic fragrances that may cause dermatitis. This simple, yet deeply hydrating body butter recipe contains essential oils that help skin look and feel amazing—without any risk of pollutants. The addition of shea butter and coconut oil promotes skin wellness and vigor.

1¾ cups shea butter

½ cup plus 2 tablespoons
   coconut oil

7 drops jasmine

7 drops vanilla absolute

⎯⎯⎯⎯

5 (4-ounce) canning jars with lids

1. In a mixing bowl, using an electric mixer on high, blend the shea butter, coconut oil, and essential oils for 6 to 8 minutes, until the mixture is smooth and has a whipped appearance.

2. Spoon into jars and use daily as needed for skin hydration.

GENTLE CLEANSING LIQUID SHAMPOO AND BODY WASH

Topical ✳ *Safe for all ages when used as directed*

Get clean while treating your skin to nurturing essential oils like lavender and chamomile. An added bonus to this combination is that it may help you and your family sleep better!

¾ cup unscented liquid castile soap

¾ cup distilled water

5 drops lavender

5 drops chamomile

———

12-ounce shampoo bottle

1. Pour the castile soap and distilled water in the bottle.

2. Add the essential oils and close the lid. Shake gently to blend.

3. Use daily in the shower or bath. Avoid contact with the eyes or mucous membranes.

COCONUT MILK SHAMPOO AND BODY WASH

Topical ✳ *Safe for all ages when used as directed*

Like coconut oil, coconut milk is a rich source of fatty acids and antioxidants. It can be a wonderful addition to your beauty routine, especially when it comes to maintaining healthy skin and hair! The addition of cedarwood and ylang-ylang maximize this recipe's hair-strengthening potential. Jojoba oil provides hair and skin with additional nutrients and softness.

½ cup unsecented liquid castile soap

⅓ cup coconut milk

2 teaspoons jojoba oil

6 drops ylang-ylang

5 drops cedarwood

2 vitamin E capsules (optional)

———

8-ounce container with lid

1. Combine the castile soap, coconut milk, and jojoba oil in the container.

2. Add the essential oils and blend thoroughly.

3. Break open two vitamin E capsules, if using, and add them to the mixture. Secure the lid and shake to blend well.

4. Use daily in the shower as both body wash and shampoo. This will keep for 1 week in the shower but will last longer if you store it in the refrigerator between uses.

HAPPY ENVIRONMENT BAR SOAP

Topical ✳ *Safe for all ages when used as directed*

If you are tired of seeing plastic everywhere, this recipe is perfect for you! Bar soap allows us to forego plastic containers and is great for those who are mindful about their impact on the environment. Bar soap lasts just as long as (or longer than) liquid soap. Clove and tangerine give this soap a powerful antibacterial punch and a lovely scent.

2 cups plus 2 tablespoons coconut oil

1 cup plus 2 tablespoons carrier oil of choice

1 cup water

4 ounces sodium hydroxide

15 drops clove

10 drops tangerine

―――――

Soap molds to make around 8 bars

1. Gently heat the coconut oil and carrier oil in a pot until melted and warmed.

2. Pour the water in a glass jar and go outdoors. Carefully add the sodium hydroxide, a tablespoon at a time, to the water. This will become very hot and put off fumes, so be careful not to inhale. Using a wood or metal spoon, gently stir until the sodium hydroxide has fully melted.

3. When the mixture has cooled, carefully add it to the warmed oils (oils should be warmed to no higher than 90 to 100°F) on the stove. Stir continuously.

4. Continue to stir and blend the ingredients together. Some people use an immersion blender off and on during this process, as they wait for the soap batter to thicken more, but this is not required as long as you stir thoroughly and continually.

Continued ➤

5. When the soap batter has thickened to "trace," it is time to add the essential oils. Trace occurs when the soap batter leaves a mark when it is drizzled across itself. When this occurs, add the essential oils and mix well.

6. Promptly pour the mixture into molds. Once the soap is in molds, leave it for 24 hours to harden. After 24 hours, remove it from the molds (slice into bars at this point, if using a mold where slicing bars is required) to cure in the open air. Let the soap cure for at least one month before using.

TIP: *Soap making is not an easy process, and it takes trial and error! Be patient and wear gloves to prevent getting any of the hot oils/ sodium hydroxide on your skin while you are making the soap. Play around with the recipe, substituting carrier and essential oils as you see fit!*

CELLULITE SMOOTHER MASSAGE BLEND

Topical ✳ *Safe for ages 15+, Phototoxic*

With astringent oils that draw and tighten skin, as well as anti-inflammatory oils, this blend can reduce the appearance of cellulite. The addition of coffee grounds exfoliates and smooths the area, and the caffeine in coffee grounds may help further reduce the appearance of cellulite.

6 drops lime

6 drops nutmeg

2 tablespoons jojoba oil

1 teaspoon ground coffee

———

1-ounce tinted glass bottle with lid

2 pipettes

1 small funnel

1. Add the essential oils to the container using pipettes.

2. Using the funnel, fill the bottle with the jojoba oil. Add the coffee, tightly secure the lid on the bottle, and shake it very well.

3. Apply a small amount to areas prone to cellulite by gently massaging in a circular motion until the oils are absorbed. You may need to dust the coffee grounds off with a towel or napkin afterward.

4. Apply this blend once daily for best results.

NOURISHING LIP BALM

Topical ✱ *Safe for ages 5+*

Two lovely and calming scents combine to create a lip balm that smells amazing and nourishes dry, cracked lips. In addition to providing healing and treatment for lips, this balm uplifts and calms the spirit.

2 tablespoons coconut oil
½ ounce beeswax pellets
1 tablespoon castor oil
15 drops vanilla absolute
10 drops lavender

───────

12 to 14 empty lip balm tubes
1 small medicine syringe

1. Bring a couple inches of water to a boil in a saucepan. Reduce the heat to maintain a simmer.

2. In a glass bowl, combine the coconut oil and beeswax pellets and place the bowl over the simmering water, stirring regularly until melted.

3. Add the castor oil and essential oils to the bowl and stir well.

4. Using the syringe, suck up the oils from the container and carefully squirt the mixture into each empty lip balm tube. This recipe should make anywhere from 12 to 14 tubes of lip balm.

5. Let the tubes sit in an undisturbed place to completely cool before using, about an hour.

6. Use this lip balm daily, or as needed for dry, cracked lips in need of nourishment.

LOVE YOUR LIPS SCRUB

Topical ✳ *Safe for ages 10+*

This lip scrub recipe is great for those with chronically dry, cracked, and chapped lips. It gently removes dead skin while providing nourishment to lips. This is an especially helpful treatment for the dry winter months.

1 tablespoon castor oil

1 tablespoon jojoba oil

3 drops helichrysum

2 to 3 tablespoons granulated sugar

8-ounce canning jar with lid

1. Add the castor oil, jojoba oil, and essential oil to the jar.

2. Add 1 tablespoon of sugar to the oils and stir, then add another tablespoon and stir again. Repeat until you have reached the desired consistency, which is usually 2 to 3 tablespoons.

3. Apply a small amount to the lips, massaging very gently. Don't scrub too hard, or you could damage your lips. Leave the treatment on for 5 to 10 minutes before rinsing it off with a warm cloth. Repeat up to three times weekly if needed.

TIP: *After using the lip scrub, try treating your lips with one of the lip balm recipes in this book. This is a great way to keep lips looking soft and supple.*

ANTIVIRAL LIP BALM FOR COLD SORES

Topical ✳ *Safe for ages 8+*

Melissa essential oil has proven antiviral properties, making it perfect for tackling cold sores before they get out of hand. When combined with other nourishing carrier oils, this lip balm will delight and heal at the same time!

2 tablespoons coconut oil
½ ounce beeswax pellets
10 drops melissa
1 tablespoon castor oil

———

12 to 14 empty lip balm tubes
1 small medicine syringe

1. Bring a couple inches of water to a boil in a saucepan. Reduce the heat to maintain a simmer.

2. In a glass bowl, combine the coconut oil and beeswax pellets and place the bowl over the simmering water, stirring regularly until melted.

3. Add the castor oil and essential oil to the bowl and stir everything well to blend.

4. Using the syringe, suck up the oils from the bowl and carefully squirt the mixture into each empty lip balm tube. This recipe should make anywhere from 12 to 14 tubes of lip balm.

5. Let the tubes sit in an undisturbed place to completely cool before using, about an hour.

6. Use this lip balm recipe at the earliest sign of a cold sore. This is most effective when used at the onset of issues.

TIP: *Another good time to use this is when your immune system is already down. For instance, when you have a cold or virus you may be more vulnerable to cold sores, so you can begin using this lip balm as a preventive measure.*

DEODORANT SPRAY

Topical ✳ *Safe for ages 10+*

Not only does lavender have a calming and lovely scent, it is highly antimicrobial. This is great if you need an oil that is gentle yet kills odor-causing bacteria. Lemongrass combines well with lavender and is also an effective antimicrobial that refreshes the skin. Colloidal silver is water that has been infused with silver particles. It can be used internally and externally to treat various infections and also kills bacteria. This is a great substitute for aluminum because it is not harmful to the body.

10 drops lavender

8 drops lemongrass

2 tablespoons vodka

3 tablespoons distilled water

1 teaspoon colloidal silver
   hydrosol

———

4-ounce tinted glass spray bottle

1 small funnel

2 pipettes

1. Add the essential oils to the bottle using pipettes.

2. Using the funnel, add the vodka, distilled water, and colloidal silver hydrosol to the bottle.

3. Screw the sprayer back on the bottle and shake vigorously before each application. Use as often as needed under the arms for odor control.

DEODORANT STICK

Topical ✳ *Safe for ages 10+*

The wonderfully aromatic essential oils in this deodorant stick blend nourish the skin while promoting sweat- and odor-free armpits! This recipe also contains other natural ingredients that are great substitutes for the synthetic ingredients in popular deodorants on the market today.

6 tablespoons coconut oil

2 tablespoons beeswax pellets

1 tablespoon shea or
   cocoa butter

¼ cup cornstarch

¼ cup aluminum-free
   baking soda

15 drops vanilla absolute

10 drops rose absolute

———

3 deodorant stick tubes

1. Bring a couple inches of water to a boil in a saucepan. Reduce the heat to maintain a simmer.

2. In a glass bowl, combine the coconut oil, beeswax, and shea butter, and place the bowl over the simmering water, stirring regularly until melted.

3. Add the cornstarch, baking soda, and essential oils to the bowl and stir them well until everything is combined.

4. Promptly pour the blend into the empty deodorant containers and let cool completely.

5. Apply under the arms up to twice daily for odor control.

TIP: *Some people are sensitive to baking soda and cornstarch. If you are one of those people, try replacing the baking soda and cornstarch with arrowroot flour.*

BALANCING TONER SPRAY

Topical ✳ *Safe for ages 15+*

This toner recipe brings balance to skin that has an uneven tone. It can restore balance and promote a healthy glow. Essential oils like clary sage and rose absolute nourish the skin and provide it with what it needs for supreme radiance.

4 drops rose absolute

3 drops clary sage

2 tablespoons distilled water

1 tablespoon witch hazel

1½ teaspoons vegetable glycerin

———

2-ounce tinted glass spray bottle

2 pipettes

1 small funnel

1. Add the essential oils to the bottle using pipettes.

2. Using the funnel, add the water, witch hazel, and vegetable glycerin to the bottle.

3. Place the sprayer back on the bottle and shake vigorously to blend. Immediately apply to the face after shaking, misting it gently with 2 to 3 sprays of toner. Shake before each use and use once daily for best results.

TIP: *Use this balancing toner after trying a clay or honey mask recipe from this book to give your skin the ultimate treat. Follow this with the Skin Brightening Serum (page 180).*

SKIN BRIGHTENING SERUM

Topical ✳ *Safe for ages 15+, Phototoxic*

A combination of lemon, basil, and chamomile can work together in this serum to enhance the luster of skin. Carrot seed oil makes the perfect carrier oil for this blend, as it may help block an enzyme that makes our skin produce melanin, which leads to skin discoloration.

6 drops chamomile
5 drops basil
4 drops lemon
2 tablespoons carrot seed oil

————

1-ounce tinted glass bottle
  with lid
3 pipettes
1 small funnel

1. Add the essential oils to the bottle using pipettes.

2. Using the funnel, fill the bottle with the carrot seed oil. Secure the lid on the bottle and shake gently to blend.

3. Apply a small amount of this serum to the face, using gentle circular motions. Lightly dab the areas around the eyes. Do not get too close to the eyes, however, because essential oils can cause burning and pain if they get in the eyes. Apply once daily at bedtime for best results.

HONEY MASK

Topical ✳ *Safe for ages 10+*

Honey is one of nature's miracles. Not only is this amazing substance great for our bodies, but it is also great for our skin! Honey is naturally antimicrobial, clearing infections and impurities when applied to the face. The addition of rose absolute and rosehip oil soothes and deeply penetrates skin in need of restoration.

1 tablespoon raw honey

½ teaspoon rosehip oil

2 drops rose absolute

1. Combine the honey, rosehip oil, and rose absolute in a small bowl.

2. Blend the ingredients together thoroughly and apply to the face.

3. Leave the mask on for 5 to 10 minutes and then rinse with warm water.

4. Apply up to three times weekly for best results.

HAIR GROWTH SERUM

Topical ✳ Safe for ages 10+

For thinning hair that breaks easily or is falling out more than usual, this serum can promote scalp circulation, as well as hair thickness and vigor. It's also a great serum for those wishing to speed up the growth of hair after a too-short haircut!

6 drops rosemary

6 drops lavender

1 tablespoon castor oil

1 tablespoon jojoba or argan oil

———

1-ounce tinted glass
   dropper bottle

2 pipettes

1 small funnel

1. Add the essential oils to the bottle using pipettes.

2. Using the funnel, add the castor oil and jojoba oil to the bottle.

3. Secure the dropper lid back on the bottle and shake the mixture well.

4. Apply a small amount to the hair, making sure to focus on the scalp.

5. Leave this serum on for 20 minutes for best results, and then rinse it out with warm water. Shampoo and wash your hair as usual. Use up to three times a week.

TIP: *To keep your hair strong and avoid breakage, pat your hair dry after getting out of the shower rather than scrubbing your head with the towel. Avoid using high heat or an abundance of products in your hair in order to prevent hair loss. Try not to wear hats either, as they can make hair fall out easier.*

HEALTHY HAIR MASK

Topical ✳ *Safe for ages 10+*

For dull hair in need of shine and luster, this mask can provide deep nourishment that penetrates into the shaft of the hair. Geranium, basil, jasmine, and ylang-ylang help keep hair healthy, strong, and radiant. Honey and vinegar rid the hair of impurities.

½ cup raw honey

2 tablespoons raw apple cider vinegar

5 drops geranium

5 drops basil

4 drops jasmine

4 drops ylang-ylang

———

8-ounce canning jar with lid

1. Combine the honey and apple cider vinegar in a container.

2. Add the essential oils to the mixture and stir well.

3. Apply this mask to the hair and leave it on for 20 minutes for best results. Rinse out thoroughly with warm water and wash your hair as usual.

HAIR DETANGLING SPRAY

Topical ✳ *Safe for ages 5+*

For thick, unruly hair that tangles easily, try this natural detangling spray for help brushing out your mane. Jojoba oil and lavender essential oil treat and prevent damage from the stress of brushing and combing, while slippery elm bark creates a natural lubricant that makes detangling easier. Apple cider vinegar promotes hair health from the inside out.

1½ cups water

4 tablespoons slippery elm bark

3 tablespoons apple
   cider vinegar

1 teaspoon jojoba oil

15 drops lavender

———

1 cheesecloth, for straining

12-ounce spray bottle

1. In a small pot, boil the water and add the slippery elm bark. Reduce the heat and let simmer for at least 20 to 30 minutes. Strain this mixture using cheesecloth set over a strainer and bowl and add it to the spray bottle.

2. Add the apple cider vinegar, jojoba oil, and lavender to the spray bottle. Secure the sprayer and shake vigorously to blend.

3. After shaking, spray evenly on towel-dried hair. Brush and repeat if necessary. Use as often as needed to help detangle and nourish unruly hair.

KILL GERMS NATURALLY LIQUID SOAP RECIPE

Topical ✽ *Safe for all ages when used as directed*

Essential oils with strong antibacterial and antiviral properties combine in this recipe to clean dirty hands. This easy, guilt-free recipe leaves hands clean and smelling warm and inviting!

¾ cup unscented liquid
   castile soap

¾ cup distilled water

5 drops cinnamon

4 drops clove

4 drops orange

_____

12-ounce liquid soap dispenser

1. Combine the castile soap and distilled water in the dispenser.

2. Add the essential oils and close the lid. Shake well to blend.

3. Apply to hands, lather, and rinse to naturally kill germs. Avoid contact with the eyes or mucous membranes.

NOURISHING MAKEUP REMOVER

Topical ✱ *Safe for ages 10+*

Rose absolute is gently astringent, evens skin tone, and clarifies. Geranium essential oil is calming to the skin and helps prevent fine lines and wrinkles. Castor oil is a great emollient, replenishing much-needed moisture to the face.

4 drops rose absolute

3 drops geranium

1 tablespoon castor oil

3 tablespoons sweet almond oil

———

2-ounce tinted glass
  dropper bottle

2 pipettes

1 small funnel

1. Add the essential oils to the bottle using pipettes.

2. Using the funnel, add the castor oil to the bottle, followed by the sweet almond oil. Secure the dropper top on the bottle and shake to mix well.

3. To use, gently wash the face with a warm washcloth.

4. Place one dropperful into your hand and gently massage it into your face, taking care to avoid getting it in the eyes. Let it sit for 1 to 2 minutes before washing it off with the washcloth.

SENSUAL PERFUME SPRAY

Topical ✳ *Safe for ages 18+*

An exotic and floral blend of jasmine, ylang-ylang, and tangerine give this intoxicating blend a dazzling twist. This combination of floral and fresh citrus aromas evokes feelings of desire and sensuality.

12 drops tangerine

10 drops ylang-ylang

10 drops jasmine

2 tablespoons vodka

———

1-ounce tinted glass spray bottle

3 pipettes

1 small funnel

1. Add the essential oils to the bottle using pipettes.

2. Using the funnel, add the vodka to the bottle.

3. Secure the sprayer on the bottle and shake vigorously to mix.

4. Spray the perfume as desired. Avoid contact with the eyes and mucous membranes. Shake the bottle before each application for a more even oil distribution.

PUMPKIN SPICE PERFUME SPRAY

Topical ✳ *Safe for ages 10+*

Fall is the perfect time to begin wearing this warm and exhilarating blend! Who doesn't love the aroma of spices used in pumpkin spice blends? This fragrance is sure to please, as well as set the mood for some fall decorating.

12 drops cinnamon

12 drops vanilla absolute

10 drops clove

10 drops nutmeg

8 drops orange

5 drops ginger

2 tablespoons vodka

———

1-ounce tinted glass spray bottle

6 pipettes

1 small funnel

1. Add the essential oils to the bottle using pipettes.

2. Using the funnel, add the vodka to the bottle.

3. Secure the sprayer on the bottle and shake vigorously to mix.

4. Spray the perfume as desired. Avoid contact with the eyes and mucous membranes. Shake the bottle before each application for a more even oil distribution.

CITRUS DREAM PERFUME SPRAY

Topical ✳ *Safe for ages 10+, Phototoxic*

A blend of stimulating and enthralling citrus essential oils create feelings of excitement and cheer. This is the perfect blend for promoting feelings of refreshment and invigoration.

12 drops tangerine

12 drops vanilla absolute

10 drops orange

10 drops lime

8 drops grapefruit

8 drops lemon

2 tablespoons vodka

———

1-ounce tinted glass spray bottle

1 small funnel

6 pipettes

1. Add the essential oils to the bottle using pipettes.

2. Using the funnel, add the vodka to the bottle.

3. Secure the sprayer on the bottle and shake vigorously to mix.

4. Spray the perfume as desired. Avoid contact with the eyes and mucous membranes. Shake the bottle before each application for a more even oil distribution.

FLORAL PERFUME SPRAY

Topical ✳ *Safe for ages 12+*

Gentle botanical aromas mingle in this floral perfume blend. The bloomy scents of jasmine, geranium, and rose combine to create a euphoric fragrance that is sure to lift your mood.

12 drops rose absolute

10 drops jasmine

10 drops geranium

2 tablespoons vodka

———

1-ounce tinted glass spray bottle

3 pipettes

1 small funnel

1. Add the essential oils to the bottle using pipettes.

2. Using the funnel, add the vodka to the bottle.

3. Secure the sprayer on the bottle and shake vigorously to mix.

4. Spray the perfume as desired. Avoid contact with the eyes and mucous membranes. Shake the bottle before each application for a more even oil distribution.

OILY SKIN TONER SPRAY

Topical ✳ *Safe for ages 10+*

For skin that is oily and acne prone, you need a toner spray that helps rid the face of bacteria that can cause acne while also removing excess oil. This recipe can help gently cleanse, replenish, and tone irritated skin.

3 drops bergamot

3 drops frankincense

2 drops basil

2 tablespoons distilled water

1 tablespoon witch hazel

1½ teaspoons vegetable glycerin

_____

2-ounce tinted glass spray bottle

3 plastic pipettes

1 small funnel

1. Add the essential oils to the bottle using pipettes.

2. Place the funnel on the bottle and add the distilled water, witch hazel, and vegetable glycerin.

3. Secure the sprayer on the bottle and shake vigorously to blend. Immediately apply 2 to 3 sprays of toner on the face after shaking. Use twice daily for best results.

TIP: *See the acne management recipes in this book for more tools to control breakouts.*

CLEANSING AND TONING CLAY MASK

Topical ✳ *Safe for ages 10+*

For skin in need of balance, this cleansing and toning clay mask can soothe, reduce redness and inflammation, and create a healthier, more even complexion. Lavender and rose oils both tone as well as nourish the skin. Bentonite clay pulls toxins and impurities from the skin.

2 tablespoons bentonite clay

1 to 2 tablespoons water

2 drops lavender

2 drops rose absolute

1. Place the bentonite clay in a small bowl. Slowly add the water, starting with only 1 tablespoon and stirring well. Keep adding a few drops of water, up to 1 tablespoon more, until a paste-like consistency is achieved.

2. Add the essential oils and stir well.

3. Apply evenly to the face and leave on for 5 to 10 minutes. Rinse off thoroughly with warm water. Repeat up to three times weekly if desired. Avoid getting this mask in the eyes.

NATURAL TOOTHPASTE RECIPE (FLUORIDE-FREE)

Topical ✳ *Safe for ages 10+*

Many commercial types of toothpaste contain controversial ingredients like artificial sweeteners, fluoride, triclosan, and sodium lauryl sulfate. If you wish to avoid these and still maintain excellent oral health, you may want to try this recipe! Clove essential oil is highly prized for its antibacterial and analgesic properties and is often indicated for issues in the mouth. Spearmint essential oil provides a refreshing and invigorating addition to this recipe. Combined, these oils will freshen breath and promote overall oral health.

½ cup coconut oil

3 tablespoons baking soda

2 natural stevia powder packets

8 drops clove

8 drops spearmint

_____

8-ounce canning jar with lid

1. Melt the coconut oil in a saucepan on low heat and transfer it to a mixing bowl.

2. Add the baking soda, stevia, and essential oils to the coconut oil. Stir thoroughly.

3. Pour the mixture in a jar for storage.

4. Use a small amount of the toothpaste twice daily. Brush normally and rinse.

TIP: *For help with remineralizing teeth, add 1 to 2 tablespoons of calcium powder to this recipe!*

HEALTHY MOUTH RINSE

Topical ✳ *Safe for ages 10+*

You don't have to turn to synthetically colorful mouthwashes for oral health. It is very easy to make your own mouthwash at home using antimicrobial essential oils like cinnamon, clove, and peppermint that also helps you maintain fresh breath.

½ cup distilled water

2 teaspoons baking soda

4 drops cinnamon

4 drops clove

3 drops peppermint

———

8-ounce canning jar with lid

1. Combine the essential oils, water, and baking soda in a jar. Secure the lid and shake well.

2. Shake well before each use. Gargle 1 to 2 tablespoons of the mouthwash for 2 to 3 minutes daily.

OIL PULLING FOR ORAL HEALTH

Topical ✳ *Safe for ages 10+*

Oil pulling is a revolutionary way to detox your mouth and body. Swishing with this blend of oils helps to get rid of surface stains, cleanse the mouth, and even protect the teeth to prevent tooth decay.

½ cup coconut oil

5 drops lemon

5 drops tea tree

―――――

4-ounce canning jar with lid

1. Melt the coconut oil and pour it into a jar.

2. Add the essential oils, secure the lid, and shake gently to blend the ingredients.

3. Swish 1 tablespoon around in your mouth daily, making sure you allow the oil to reach all parts of the mouth. Swish for a total of 10 minutes before spitting the oil out into the trash. Never swallow this oil mixture, as it pulls out toxins from the body.

4. Try oil pulling daily, or every other day, for best results.

TIP: *For young children, skip the essential oils and have them use only coconut oil for oil pulling.*

STRETCH MARK AND SCAR ROLLER REMEDY

Topical ✳ *Safe for ages 10+*

Stretch marks are a type of scar on the skin that forms when the body goes through swift growth. Oftentimes, pregnancy and adolescence can bring on stretch marks. Skin nourishing oils combine in this remedy to treat skin in need of healing, replenishment, and restoration. They provide balance and toning to stretch marks and scars, as well as improve circulation to the area. Jojoba oil makes a good carrier oil for this blend because of its gentle, skin-mending properties.

10 drops helichrysum

5 drops jasmine

4 drops cypress

4 drops patchouli

1 tablespoon jojoba oil

———

½-ounce (15 ml) tinted glass roller bottle

4 pipettes

1 small funnel

1. Add the essential oils to the roller bottle using pipettes.

2. Using the funnel, fill the bottle with the jojoba oil. Place the roller and cap on the bottle and shake well.

3. Apply this blend to problem areas up to twice daily for best results.

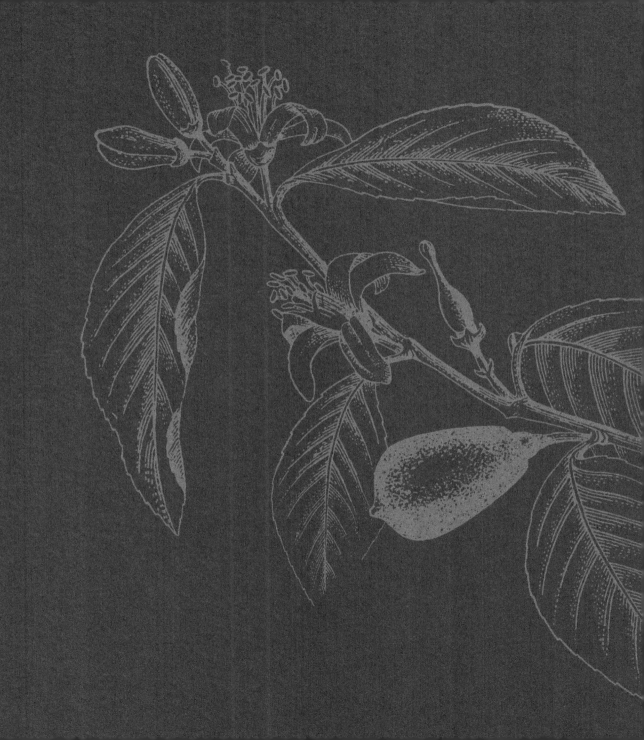

CHAPTER EIGHT

Home and Outdoors

The great thing about essential oils is that although they can be gentle and natural, they are also powerful and have the ability to kill bacteria and viruses and cut through grime. They make an excellent choice for replacing everyday household cleaning products that may contain lethal ingredients. In this chapter, you will learn how to use essential oils for cleaning your carpet, windows, grout, shower, toilet bowl, washing machine, garbage disposal, and even your car!

BANISH BAD SMELLS DIFFUSION BLEND

Diffusion ✳ *Safe for ages 10+*

Without good ventilation, unpleasant smells can seem to set in and never leave. This blend not only helps purify the air, but also makes your house smell nice and refreshing! The oils in this blend work together to neutralize bad odors instead of just hiding them.

4 drops clove

4 drops lemon

2 drops ravensara

———

1 ultrasonic diffuser

1. Fill the diffuser with water up to the water line. Add the essential oils to the diffuser.

2. Turn it on and let the diffuser run until it is out of water.

TIP: *Since clove essential oil is a "hot" oil, it is advised to diffuse this blend when no children are present to avoid any reactions.*

REENERGIZING ROOM SPRAY

Diffusion ✳ *Safe for ages 10+*

Liven up a stale room with this blend of aromatic essential oils! Together, they uplift, invigorate, and provide a stimulating and refreshing atmosphere.

10 drops tangerine

8 drops peppermint

2 drops rosemary

¼ cup distilled water

———

2-ounce tinted glass spray bottle

3 pipettes

1 small funnel

1. Add the essential oils to the spray bottle using pipettes.

2. Using the funnel, add the distilled water to the bottle, leaving room for the sprayer to be inserted. Secure the sprayer on the bottle and shake well before spraying.

3. Spray in the air and not directly onto surfaces. Try this once a day, or as needed, to reenergize a room. Shake the bottle before each application for more even oil distribution.

TIP: *Since this blend contains rosemary and peppermint, it should not be used around children under the age of ten due to the constituent 1,8-cineole, which can cause respiratory issues.*

WARM AND INVITING WAX MELT RECIPE

Diffusion ✻ *Safe for ages 5+ years (safe for occasional inhalation, but not to touch)*

There is nothing like walking into a home that smells hospitable and welcoming! People spend a lot of money on products with synthetic fragrances to help their home smell better, but the truth is that these products may cause more harm than good. Many synthetic fragrances can cause migraines, respiratory issues, and worse. This blend of essential oils will create an atmosphere of warmth and coziness in your home. When combined, they make the perfect fragrance for holidays, or times when families gather.

½ cup soy wax pellets

¼ cup coconut oil

20 drops cinnamon

20 drops vanilla absolute

10 drops orange

———

1 silicone mold with several small, 1-inch cavities

1 wax melter

1. Bring a few inches of water to a boil in a saucepan. Reduce the heat to maintain a simmer.

2. Combine the soy wax pellets and coconut oil in a glass measuring cup or bowl and set the cup in the simmering water until completely melted.

3. Add the essential oils. Using a wooden or metal spoon, stir well.

4. Quickly (but not too quickly) pour the oil and wax mixture into the silicone mold and let it cool completely.

5. Store the wax melts in a cool place. Add one to a wax melter to scent your home.

REFRESHING AND UPLIFTING WAX MELT RECIPE

Diffusion ✳ *Safe for ages 10+*

What better way to provide your home with a positively energizing aroma than with citrus essential oils? Grapefruit and tangerine essential oils are both uplifting and mood-boosting. They promote a sense of optimism and elevation. Peppermint enhances these oils by adding a gently stimulating and invigorating aspect to their synergy. When combined in a rousing blend, they completely transform a dull room.

½ cup soy wax pellets

¼ cup coconut oil

20 drops tangerine

20 drops grapefruit

7 drops peppermint

———

1 silicone mold with several small, 1-inch cavities

1 wax melter

1. Bring a few inches of water to a boil in a saucepan. Reduce the heat to maintain a simmer.

2. Combine the soy wax pellets and coconut oil in a glass measuring cup or bowl and set the cup in the simmering water until completely melted.

3. Add the essential oils. Using a wooden or metal spoon, stir well.

4. Quickly (but not too quickly) pour the oil and wax mixture into the silicone mold and let it cool completely.

5. Store the wax melts in a cool place. Add one to a wax melter to scent your home.

PILLOW AND SHEET SPRAY

Diffusion ✳ *Safe for ages 5+*

Lavender and chamomile are some of the most popular oils for helping the body relax and fall asleep. They are also antimicrobial and may kill any bacteria lurking on your bedsheets. Try this recipe and let these oils pull double duty in your bed.

10 drops chamomile
10 drops lavender
2 tablespoons distilled water

———

1-ounce tinted glass spray bottle
2 pipettes
1 small funnel

1. Add the essential oils to the bottle using pipettes.

2. Using the funnel, add the water to the bottle.

3. Secure the sprayer on the bottle and shake vigorously to blend.

4. After shaking, spray onto bedsheets and pillowcases at least 2 hours before bedtime. Do this nightly to maintain clean sheets and promote a good night's sleep.

BUG BITE SOOTHING ROLLER BLEND

Topical ✴ *Safe for ages 5+*

Sometimes, no matter what you do, bugs still find a way to bite. This is where essential oils come in handy. They can help soothe irritated, red skin as well as control the histamine reaction caused by the bug bite.

15 drops tea tree

15 drops lavender

1 tablespoon carrier oil of choice

———

½-ounce (15 ml) tinted glass roller bottle

2 pipettes

1 small funnel

1. Add the essential oils to the bottle using pipettes.

2. Using the funnel, fill the bottle with the carrier oil. Place the roller and cap on the bottle and shake well.

3. Apply directly to bug bites up to three times daily to help control itching and discomfort.

TICK BITE RESCUE ROLLER BLEND

Topical ✳ *Safe for ages 10+*

Tick bites come with their own set of issues. With all the different tick-borne illnesses today, it is important to keep a close eye on tick bites, as well as treat the area with essential oils that kill viruses and bacteria while promoting skin healing.

6 drops geranium

4 drops cinnamon

3 drops thyme

1 tablespoon carrier oil of choice

———

½-ounce (15 ml) tinted glass roller bottle

3 pipettes

1 small funnel

1. Add the essential oils to the bottle using pipettes.

2. Using the funnel, fill the bottle with the carrier oil. Place the roller and cap on the bottle and shake well.

3. Apply directly to tick bites as soon as the tick is removed. Continue to treat once daily.

TIP: *After discovering a tick bite, remove it safely with tick twisters instead of tweezers, which may cause the tick to vomit inside you and release toxic substances. You may choose to keep the tick and send it off for testing. Keep a close eye on the bite, looking for any red ring around the area (referred to as a "bullseye"), and pay attention to how you feel. If you begin to feel fatigued, run a low-grade fever, or have any other suspicious symptoms, see a medical professional immediately.*

CAR REFRESH SPRAY

Diffusion ✳ *Safe for all ages when used as directed*

Lemongrass has a refreshing and revitalizing aroma. When paired with tangerine, it enlivens the stale air inside a car. Lavender adds a hint of floral aroma and helps to eliminate bacteria that cause unwanted smells. When combined, these oils can both neutralize and replace car odors with energizing aromas.

8 drops tangerine

5 drops lemongrass

5 drops lavender

2 tablespoons vodka

3 tablespoons distilled water

4-ounce tinted glass spray bottle

3 pipettes

1 small funnel

1. Add the essential oils to the glass bottle using pipettes.

2. Using the funnel, add the vodka and distilled water to the bottle.

3. Secure the sprayer on the bottle. Shake vigorously before spraying in your car.

4. Spray throughout the car and gently wipe down with a cloth if any drops are left on seats, the steering wheel, etc. Don't forget to liberally spray the floorboards!

TIP: *Be cautious of applying this spray on upholstered or leather seats until you do a small spot check to make sure no discoloration will occur.*

GARBAGE DISPOSAL CLEANER

Cleaner ✳ *Safe for all ages when used as directed*

A powerful blend of citrus essential oils helps to clean the garbage disposal, as well as promote an invigorating and refreshing aroma in the kitchen.

4 tablespoons salt
15 drops lemon
10 drops grapefruit
1 cup ice

1. Begin the process by making sure nothing is down in the garbage disposal, using tongs to remove stuck objects, etc.

2. Next, run hot water to help break down residual grease. Let it run a minute or two and then shut the water off.

3. In a small bowl, combine the salt and essential oils.

4. Toss the salt and oil combination in with the ice cubes and mix as well as you can.

5. Place the mixture down in the garbage disposal (make sure it is not running).

6. Turn on the garbage disposal and let it break up the ice and salt. Turn on cold water to continue the cleaning process as the garbage disposal runs.

7. Turn off the garbage disposal when the ice is eliminated. Scrub it with a brush to further clean the area.

TIP: *When finished, add a few lemon peels or 5 to 10 drops of lemon essential oil to the garbage disposal to ensure cleanliness and a wonderful aroma!*

ATTRACT POLLINATORS TO YOUR GARDEN

Diffusion ✳ *Safe for all ages when used as directed*

Although essential oils are widely used to repel bugs, some essential oils can actually attract bugs—the good kind, that is! Attract pollinators to your garden with lemongrass and marjoram to promote vibrant, beautiful plants.

12 drops lemongrass

12 drops marjoram

———

2 small cloths

2 strings or pieces of yarn

1. Apply lemongrass essential oil to one cloth, dripping in different places on the cloth.

2. Apply marjoram essential oil to another cloth, dripping in different places on the cloth.

3. Tie each cloth to a string and hang them in areas of your garden where you want to attract pollinators like honeybees and butterflies. Repeat this monthly for best results.

APHID-REPELLANT SPRAY

*Diffusion * Safe for all ages when used as directed*

Aphids can destroy vegetables in your garden that you put time and effort into growing. Repel these unwanted garden guests with spearmint and cedarwood essential oils!

12 drops spearmint

12 drops cedarwood

3 tablespoons plus
  1½ teaspoons distilled water

———

2-ounce tinted glass spray bottle

1 small funnel

2 pipettes

1. Add the essential oils to the bottle using pipettes.

2. Using the funnel, add the distilled water to the bottle. Secure the sprayer on the bottle and shake well before spraying.

3. Lightly mist the areas where aphids tend to congregate on your garden plants. Do this daily to help repel aphids.

TIP: *Another great and natural way to get rid of aphids is to order ladybugs and release them in your garden!*

SLUG AND SNAIL REPELLANT SPRAY

Diffusion ✳ *Safe for all ages when used as directed*

Slugs and snails can do a lot of damage for such small creatures. They love to dine on plants like cabbage and lettuce. Because these plants have such long growing seasons, they are exposed to a variety of pests. Help keep them pest-free with pine and patchouli essential oils!

10 drops pine

10 drops patchouli

3 tablespoons plus

1½ teaspoons ounces
   distilled water

———

2-ounce tinted glass spray bottle

1 small funnel

2 pipettes

1. Add the essential oils to the bottle using pipettes.

2. Using the funnel, add the distilled water to the bottle. Secure the sprayer on the bottle and shake well before spraying.

3. Lightly mist the vegetables snails and slugs like to eat. Do this daily to keep them at bay.

GET GROUT CLEAN

Cleaner ✳ *Safe for all ages when used as directed*

Lemon and tea tree essential oils are a great cleansing combination. Vinegar is also antibacterial and an excellent base for any cleaning product. Baking soda provides an alkaline agent to the mixture that also acts as an exfoliator. Combining these two popular essential oils with vinegar and baking soda helps make even the dirtiest grout shine.

6 drops lemon

5 drops tea tree

2 tablespoons baking soda

3 tablespoons distilled
white vinegar

———

2-ounce tinted glass spray bottle

2 pipettes

1 small funnel

1 old toothbrush or small
scrubber

1. Add the essential oils to the bottle using pipettes.

2. Using the funnel, add the baking soda and vinegar to the bottle. When adding the baking soda, you may need to tap it a few times to get it through the funnel.

3. Secure the sprayer on the bottle and shake it very well before spraying on the surfaces you want to clean.

4. If cleaning grout on the floors, sweep the floor very thoroughly before beginning. If cleaning grout on the walls, wipe with a warm, wet cloth before beginning.

5. Spray the grout cleaner on the desired areas and let it sit for 10 to 15 minutes before gently scrubbing with a brush.

6. When finished, wipe everything down with a warm, wet cloth.

MOLD KILLER DIFFUSION BLEND

Diffusion ✱ *Safe for ages 10+*

This protocol can help eliminate mold caused by dampness in an area of your home. To get to the root of the problem, make sure the cause of the dampness is addressed. It is also advisable to purchase a dehumidifier to use in conjunction with this diffusion blend.

8 drops tea tree

3 drops clove

3 drops lavender

———

1 ultrasonic diffuser

1. Fill the diffuser with water up to the water line. Add the essential oils to the diffuser.

2. Turn it on and let the diffuser run until it is empty. Do this daily for mold control.

TIP: *After running the diffuser, eliminate excess water from the room by running a dehumidifier.*

SAY BYE TO BUGS BODY SPRAY

Topical ✻ *Safe for ages 6+*

Going for a hike or preparing to spend some time outdoors? This body spray may be the perfect bug repellant for you! A combination of citronella, lemongrass, and lavender will repel a variety of bugs, from mosquitoes to ticks.

10 drops citronella

10 drops lemongrass

8 drops lavender

3 tablespoons plus

1½ teaspoons distilled water

———

2-ounce tinted glass spray bottle

3 plastic pipettes

1 small funnel

1. Add the essential oils to the bottle using pipettes.

2. Using the funnel, add the distilled water to the bottle.

3. Secure the sprayer on the bottle and shake vigorously before applying to the clothes and body.

4. Apply up to three times daily, as needed, for protection from insects like mosquitoes, ticks, and chiggers.

BUG-REPELLANT SOY WAX CANDLE

Diffusion ✳ *Safe for all ages when used outdoors as directed*

This handmade citronella candle recipe is great for use outdoors. It can repel mosquitoes and other bothersome insects so you can enjoy time outdoors on your deck!

---

440 grams soy wax pellets

20 to 30 drops citronella

———

16-ounce glass jar

1 tall wick

Hot glue gun

1. At the bottom of the glass jar, glue a wick using the hot glue gun and set it aside. Let it dry completely. You can help keep the wick in place as it dries by wrapping the top around a small stick, spoon, or related object that can sit across the top of the jar.

2. Fill a large pot about one-third full of water and bring it to a boil. Reduce the heat and simmer.

3. Place the soy wax into a smaller pot and sit this pot inside the large pot of water. Be careful not to splash any hot water on yourself.

4. Allow the soy wax to melt completely. Add the citronella and mix well.

5. Pour the mixture into the candle jar and allow it to cool. Keep the wick in place and trim to your desired length when finished drying.

6. Burn this candle where you are spending time outdoors to repel mosquitoes.

KEEP FLEAS OUT DOOR AND FOUNDATION SPRAY

Cleaning ✳ *Safe for all ages when used as directed*

Fleas can become a problem in the summer months when the weather is warming up. In the fall, they can become even worse, as they tend to multiply swiftly during these months. Without proper prevention, fleas can become a major problem in a house. Repel them from your home with a combination of citronella, peppermint, and eucalyptus.

20 drops citronella

20 drops peppermint

20 drops eucalyptus

1¼ cups plus 2 tablespoons distilled water

———————

12-ounce tinted spray bottle

1. Add the distilled water to the spray bottle.

2. Add the essential oils to the water and secure the lid tightly.

3. Shake vigorously and apply this spray to the doorframes and foundation of your home daily to prevent flea infestations. Shake well before each use to distribute the oils and store in a cool, dry place for up to 2 years.

TIP: *If you are a pet owner, caution is advised when using essential oils around your pet. Many pets respond differently to oils than humans and can have a harder time processing them. Use this spray outdoors only if you have indoor pets. If you have outdoor pets, keep them away from the areas you spray until it is completely dry.*

CARPET POWDER FOR ODOR NEUTRALIZATION

Cleaner ✱ *Safe for all ages when used as directed*

A mixture of antimicrobial essential oils to target odor-causing bacteria, as well as purifying oils to deep clean, makes this carpet powder a winner! Baking soda is the base for this formula because it is known for its ability to combat unwanted smells.

1 (8-ounce) box baking soda

10 drops lavender

6 drops tea tree

6 drops tangerine

———

8-ounce canning jar with holes in lid for sprinkling

1. Pour the baking soda into a mixing bowl. Add the essential oils to the baking soda. Stir the mixture until it is well blended.

2. Transfer the mixture to the canning jar and screw the sprinkling lid on.

3. When you encounter a pet mess, soak up as much as possible first using a thick towel. Wash the area with soapy water and let it dry for a few hours.

4. Liberally sprinkle the carpet powder on the affected area (rub it into the fibers of the carpet as well) and let this sit overnight if possible.

5. Vacuum the area the next day and repeat application, if necessary, until the smell is gone.

TIP: *Always test a small spot to make sure there will be no discoloration before applying this powder to a large area. Store the powder in a cool, dry place and replace the shaker lid with one that does not have holes to keep it fresh. This will last for as long as the expiration on the baking soda you purchase indicates.*

POISON IVY PROTECTION BLEND

Topical ✳ *Safe for ages 6+*

If you are outdoors much, you are probably aware of the dangers of plants like poison ivy, poison sumac, and poison oak. This blend can help protect your skin from exposure to the urushiol found on the leaves of these plants. Geranium and lavender essential oils care for the skin and a protectant carrier oil like avocado oil forms a barrier, diluting any urushiol that may come into contact with the skin.

8 drops geranium
8 drops lavender
¼ cup avocado oil

———

2-ounce jar with lid

1. Add the essential oils to the jar.

2. Add the avocado oil to the jar and secure the lid. Gently shake to mix the oils.

3. Apply a liberal amount of this blend to exposed skin before going outdoors.

4. When returning home, shower immediately to wash off any toxic oils using a grease-cutting soap. Scrub the skin with a washcloth as you wash your skin to further aid in ridding the skin of any problematic plant oils.

SANITIZING SPRAY FOR HANDS AND SURFACES

Topical, Cleaner ✻ *Safe for ages 10+*

Blending oils that kill germs and bacteria, as well as oils that are antifungal and cleansing, make this an effective sterilizer.

4 drops tea tree

3 drops orange

2 drops clove

2 drops cinnamon

2 tablespoons vodka

3 tablespoons distilled water

———

2-ounce tinted glass spray bottle

1 small funnel

4 pipettes

1. Add the essential oils in the bottle using pipettes.

2. Using the funnel, add the vodka and distilled water to the bottle.

3. Secure the sprayer on the bottle and shake vigorously before applying. Spray away from the eyes.

4. If using on hands, apply one pump of spray to each hand and rub them together well. Spray on nonporous surfaces like the table at a restaurant to help clean where you will be eating.

TIP: *For a kid-safe version of this blend, leave out clove and cinnamon and replace the vodka with vegetable glycerin.*

SANITIZING WIPES

Topical ✳ *Safe for ages 10+*

Another great way to enjoy sanitizing essential oils is to create sanitizing wipes. These make it even easier to disinfect surfaces and hands!

¾ cup distilled water

¾ cup rubbing alcohol

6 drops lavender

5 drops clove

5 drops lemongrass

———————

Recycled cloth pieces, for use as wipes

16-ounce glass canning jar with lid

1. Add the distilled water, rubbing alcohol, and essential oils to the glass jar. Place the lid on the jar and shake it well to mix.

2. Stuff as many small pieces of cloth as you can fit into the jar. Leave an inch or so of room at the top. Close the lid.

3. Gently turn the bottle upside down and back up again to get the liquid to saturate into all of the wipes.

4. Grab a wipe from the jar as needed to clean hands and surfaces. Carry this in the car for when you are on the go or leave it on the counter to help clean up. The wipes can be reused after washing for a waste-free solution to cleaning!

REMOVE THE MARK BLEND

Cleaner ✳ *Safe for all ages when used as directed*

Depending on the object used to create the mark, marks on walls and furniture can be stubborn and hard to remove. Lemon and lime essential oils break down substances in markers and can gently remove marks and scuffs around the house. This combination works well on solid surfaces like floors, walls, and countertops.

---

1 drop lemon
1 drop lime

1. Combine the essential oils in a small container and then dip a cloth into the oils.

2. Gently apply this to the mark. Leave it on for 1 to 2 minutes before gently scrubbing with the cloth to remove the mark.

3. Rinse the area with soapy water and dry thoroughly when finished.

TIP: *Always perform a patch test on a small area before applying any essential oils. This will help you determine whether or not the oils may react with a paint or stain and cause discoloration.*

SHOWER REFRESHING SPRAY

Cleaner ✳ *Safe for all ages when used as directed*

Lime and lavender essential oils can help combat mold and mildew lurking in the corners of your shower. This refreshing and useful shower spray recipe cleanses and protects your shower without the use of synthetic chemicals.

10 drops lime

5 drops lavender

¼ cup white distilled vinegar

_____

2-ounce tinted glass spray bottle

1 small funnel

2 pipettes

1. Add the essential oils to the bottle using pipettes.

2. Using the funnel, add the vinegar to the bottle. Secure the sprayer on the bottle and shake the mixture vigorously before spraying in the shower.

3. Keep this solution in your shower and spray the walls around you, as well as all nooks and crannies, every time you finish showering to help prevent and combat scum, mold, and mildew.

ALL-PURPOSE VINEGAR CLEANER

Cleaner ✳ *Safe for use on nonporous surfaces in the home*

This combination of essential oils can clean, disinfect, and provide a lustrous sheen to household surfaces, making it an invaluable blend. The citrus oils also smell wonderful and can promote an uplifted mood as you clean the house! Vinegar is a staple in most homes, and although it is often used in cooking, it can also be used to clean.

20 drops lemon

20 drops orange

2 cups white distilled vinegar

2 cups water

——————

1-quart spray bottle

2 plastic pipettes

1 funnel

1. Add the essential oils to the spray bottle using pipettes.

2. Using the funnel, add the vinegar and water to the bottle.

3. Secure the sprayer on the bottle and shake it very well before spraying the cleaner on nonporous surfaces.

4. The oil and vinegar will not mix well, but if you shake it before applying it to surfaces, it will distribute fine. After spraying, wipe the area with a clean cloth.

TIP: *Avoid using this mixture on granite or other stone surfaces.*

TOILET BOWL SPRAY

Cleaner ✳ *Safe for all ages when used as directed*

The essential oils in this recipe cut through grime and kill germs. The addition of vinegar, baking soda, and salt help scrub away unwanted stains in the toilet bowl.

1 cup white distilled vinegar

20 drops lemon, divided

20 drops clove, divided

1 cup baking soda

¼ cup salt

_____

8-ounce canning jar with holes in lid for sprinkling

8-ounce spray container

1. Add the vinegar and 10 drops of each essential oil to the spray container and set it aside.

2. Add the baking soda, salt, and 10 drops of each essential oil to the canning jar and mix well.

3. Shake the vinegar and essential oil spray bottle well and spray all over the inside of the toilet bowl.

4. Immediately begin sprinkling the areas you just sprayed with the baking soda mixture as well. You may notice a fizzing sound as a result.

5. Let the cleaner sit undisturbed for at least 20 to 40 minutes, then scrub the bowl thoroughly with a toilet brush. Flush the toilet and repeat if necessary.

WASHING MACHINE REFRESH BLEND

Cleaner ✳ *Safe for all ages when used as directed*

To kill the germs responsible for the odors coming from a washing machine, antimicrobial and antifungal essential oils are needed. The oils in this recipe eliminate unwanted smells, as well as mold and mildew.

10 drops tea tree

10 drops lavender

5 drops eucalyptus

1 cup distilled white vinegar

––––––––

8-ounce canning jar with lid

1. Add the essential oils and vinegar to a jar.

2. Close the lid of the jar and shake to distribute evenly, or if you do not have a lid, stir the solution. Immediately add this mixture to the washing machine when it is full of hot water (and nothing else).

3. Run the washing machine through a normal cycle with only the water and cleaning solution.

4. When the cycle is over, use a cloth to wipe down the inside of the machine, making sure to wipe around the seal, door, and drum. Let the washing machine dry completely before running it with clothes inside.

NATURAL WINDOW CLEANING TREATMENT

Cleaner ✳ *Safe for all ages when used as directed*

The vibrant and invigorating essential oils in this recipe create a light, refreshing atmosphere while leaving a streak-free, clean surface on glass. This spray can be used on mirrors and windows in the home, as well as car windows.

2 cups distilled or
  reverse-osmosis water

¼ cup distilled white vinegar

¼ cup rubbing alcohol

1 tablespoon cornstarch

10 drops bergamot

10 drops lime

———

18-ounce spray bottle

1. Pour the water, vinegar, and rubbing alcohol into the spray bottle.

2. Add the cornstarch and essential oils and secure the sprayer on the bottle.

3. Shake the mixture thoroughly and lightly spray onto surfaces. Use a dry cloth to wipe the surfaces clean.

4. Shake before each use to properly distribute the oils. Store in a cool, dry place for up to 2 years.

GLOSSARY OF AROMATHERAPY TERMS

These common terms describing properties of essential oils will help you decide which essential oil provides the benefits you're looking for.

Absolute: alcohol-based essential oil extract with 5 to 10 parts per million of solvent residue remaining from the extraction process

Adulterated: oil containing anything other than pure, 100 percent essential oil

Analgesic: relieves pain

Anesthetic: relieves pain or offers a numbing effect

Anti-allergenic: prevents histamine reaction that leads to allergies

Anti-infectious: capable of acting against infection, either by inhibiting the spread of an infectious agent or by killing the infectious agent outright

Anti-inflammatory: prevents or reduces inflammation

Antibacterial: fights bacterial growth

Antibiotic: destroys bacteria or prevents its growth

Antidepressant: provides relief from symptoms of depression

Antifungal: prevents fungal growth

Antimicrobial: kills microorganisms or inhibits their growth

Antineuralgic: relieves nerve pain

Antioxidant: inhibits oxidation

Antiparasitic: kills parasites

Antiphlogistic: counteracting inflammation and/or a feverish state

Antiseptic: controls infection

Antispasmodic: prevents cramping and/or muscle spasms

Antitumoral: inhibits the growth of tumors

Antiviral: fights viral infections

Astringent: encourages tissues to tighten

Bactericidal: kills bacteria

Bulking: using plants from the same species but from different harvests to reduce the cost of a specific oil

Carminative: facilitates healthy digestion and prevents gas formation in the digestive tract

Decongestant: relieves congestion

Digestive: aids in digestion

Disinfectant: destroys, neutralizes, or inhibits the growth of disease-carrying micro-organisms

Emmenagogue: stimulates or promotes menstruation

Emollient: softens skin

Energizing: promotes vitality and energy

Euphoric: promotes feelings of happiness

Expectorant: encourages the elimination of mucus

Febrifuge: fever reducer

Fungicide: kills fungus

Hemostatic: stops or prevents bleeding

Hypertensive: causes an increase in blood pressure

Hypotensive: causes a decrease in blood pressure

Immunostimulant: stimulates the immune system

Insecticide: kills insects

Nervine: acts upon the nerves to quiet nervous tension or excitement

Sanitizing: to make sanitary by sterilizing

Sedative: promotes or enhances relaxation; may induce sleep

Stimulant: promotes or enhances alertness

Stomachic: stimulates digestion or strengthens the stomach

Recommended Essential Oil Brands

Please be aware when shopping that all of the brands listed below sell both organic and non-organic essential oils.

BRAND	PROS	CONS
PLANT THERAPY *planttherapy.com*	✳ A big line of organic oils to choose from ✳ A line of kid-safe essential oils ✳ Reasonably priced	✳ Some of their kid-safe blends do not call for enough dilution
MOUNTAIN ROSE HERBS *mountainroseherbs.com*	✳ Large line of organic essential oils ✳ Lots of information about their products on their website	✳ Slightly more expensive than other companies ✳ Safety information is not as detailed
AURA CACIA *auracacia.com*	✳ A decent-sized line of organic oils ✳ Affordable	✳ No GC/MS reports available on their website
ARTISAN AROMATICS *artisanaromatics.com*	✳ A line of sustainably wildcrafted essential oils ✳ Offers a decent selection of oils	✳ Pricey
EDEN BOTANICALS *edenbotanicals.com*	✳ Offers a wide array of organic oils ✳ Offers several size options	✳ Pricey

REFERENCES

Agricultural Marketing Service. "Organic Certification and Accreditation." Accessed September 2019. https://www.ams.usda.gov/services/organic-certification.

Al-Yasiry, Ali Ridha Mustafa, and Bożena Kiczorowska. "Frankincense—Therapeutic Properties." *Postępy Higieny i Medycyny Doświadczalnej (Advances in Hygiene and Experimental Medicine)* (Online). U.S. National Library of Medicine, January 4, 2016. https://www.ncbi.nlm.nih.gov/pubmed/27117114.

Aromahead Institute. "The Aromahead Blog - Aromatherapy Education and Resources." Accessed September 2019. https://blog.aromahead.com.

AromaWeb. Accessed September 2019. https://www.aromaweb.com.

Bowles, E. Joy. *The Chemistry of Aromatherapeutic Oils*. Crows Nest, Australia: Allen & Unwin, 2004.

Butje, Andrea. *The Heart of Aromatherapy: An Easy-to-Use Guide for Essential Oils*. Carlsbad, CA: Hay House, 2017.

DavidWolfe (blog). "Study: Smelling Rosemary Increases Memory By 75%." Accessed September 23, 2019. https://www.davidwolfe.com/study-claims-smelling-rosemary-increases-memory-by-75.

Harding, Jennie. The *Essential Oils Handbook: All the Oils You Will Ever Need for Health, Vitality and Well-Being*. London: Watkins Publishing, 2018.

Koulivand, Peir Hossein, Maryam Khaleghi Ghadiri, and Ali Gorji. "Lavender and the Nervous System." *Evidence-Based Complementary and Alternative Medicine*. 2013. doi:10.1155/2013/681304.

Lawless, Julia. *The Encyclopedia of Essential Oils*. Rockport, MA: Element Books Ltd., 1996.

National Association for Holistic Aromatherapy. Accessed September 2019. https://naha.org.

Price, Len, and Shirley Price. *Carrier Oils for Aromatherapy and Massage*. Stratford-upon-Avon, UK: Riverhead, 2008.

Schnaubelt, Kurt. *Advanced Aromatherapy: The Science of Essential Oil Therapy*. Rochester, VT: Healing Arts Press, 1998.

Schnaubelt, Kurt. *The Healing Intelligence of Essential Oils: The Science of Advanced Aromatherapy.* Rochester, VT: Healing Arts Press, 2011.

Tisserand, Robert, and Tony Balacs. *Essential Oil Safety: A Guide For Health Care Professionals.* London: Churchill Livingstone Elsevier, 2000.

Tisserand, Robert. *The Art of Aromatherapy.* Saffron Walden, UK: The C. W. Daniel Company Ltd, 2009.

Tisserand Institute. "Robert Tisserand Interviewed on Ingestion, Dilution and Other Safety Issues." Accessed April 24, 2018. https://roberttisserand.com/2015/08/robert-tisserand-interviewed-on-ingestion-dilution-and-other-safety-issues.

Tyko, Kelly. "Man Awarded $80M in Lawsuit Claiming Monsanto's Roundup Causes Cancer." USA Today. Accessed March 28, 2019. https://www.usatoday.com/story/money/2019/03/27/monsanto-roundup-cancer-lawsuit-california-man-awarded-80-million/3293824002.

Using Essential Oils Safely (blog). "Using Essential Oils Safely | Know Better, Do Better." Accessed September 2019. https://www.usingeossafely.com.

Worwood, Valerie Ann. *The Complete Book of Essential Oils and Aromatherapy: Over 800 Natural, Nontoxic, and Fragrant Recipes to Create Health, Beauty, and Safe Home and Work Environments.* Novato, CA: New World Library, 2016.

INDEX

ABOUT THE AUTHOR

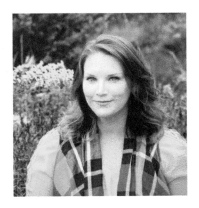

Amber Robinson is a NAHA Level 2 Professional Aromatherapist, as well as an AHG Registered Herbalist. She works with essential oils in an intimate way, teaching the craft of essential oil distillation at her school, The Bitter Herb Academy.

Amber enjoys growing, wildcrafting, and harvesting plants on her farm in the Missouri Ozarks, which she uses to create her own essential oils. She is a wife and mother of two little boys, and loves spending her days teaching them, as well as her students, about essential oils and plant medicine.